A CAMPAIGN AGAINST
CONSUMPTION

A CAMPAIGN AGAINST CONSUMPTION

A COLLECTION OF PAPERS RELATING TO TUBERCULOSIS

BY

ARTHUR RANSOME, M.D., F.R.C.P., F.R.S.

Hon. Fellow of Caius College, Cambridge ;
Consulting Physician to the Manchester Hospital for Consumption,
and to the Bournemouth Hospital ;
Late Professor of Public Health to Victoria University and Examiner in
Sanitary Science and Public Health to Cambridge and Victoria Universities ;
Milroy Lecturer to Royal College of Physicians (in 1890)

" Rally the scattered causes, and the line
That nature twists, be ready to untwine."

Religio Medici.

Cambridge :

at the University Press

1915

CAMBRIDGE
UNIVERSITY PRESS

University Printing House, Cambridge CB2 8BS, United Kingdom

Published in the United States of America by Cambridge University Press, New York

Cambridge University Press is part of the University of Cambridge.

It furthers the University's mission by disseminating knowledge in the pursuit of education, learning and research at the highest international levels of excellence.

www.cambridge.org
Information on this title: www.cambridge.org/9781107418998

© Cambridge University Press 1915

First published 1915
First paperback edition 2014

A catalogue record for this publication is available from the British Library

ISBN 978-1-107-41899-8 Paperback

TO

THE MEMORY OF MY GRANDFATHER

JOHN ATKINSON RANSOME, F.R.C.S.

WHO FIRST PROPOSED, AND MADE USE OF, ANIMAL GUT
IN THE LIGATURE OF ARTERIES

AND OF MY FATHER

JOSEPH ATKINSON RANSOME, F.R.C.S.

WHO FIRST USED CARBOLIC ACID IN THE TREATMENT
OF SEPTIC WOUNDS

PREFACE

I HAVE been engaged in fighting against CONSUMPTION for more than 50 years, and have been urged to re-publish, in book form, some of my writings which deal with the subject from a public health point of view, and others which take a more purely scientific form.

In the present volume, therefore, are brought together a number of Papers relating to Tuberculosis. Most of them have been read before various Societies, such as the Royal Society, the Epidemiological Society, the Sanitary Institute, and the National Association for the Prevention of Tuberculosis, etc., and have appeared in their Transactions, or in Medical Journals. Others again have been separately published, but are now out of print, and, probably, out of mind.

At the present time, much attention is being given to the subject of the prevention of the disease; and the Papers are now therefore re-printed, partly as a contribution to the history of the movement, but mainly in the hope that they may still help in the furtherance of this object.

My own entrance into the campaign against consumption dates back to the year 1860, when I was able to start in Manchester and Salford a weekly Register of all new cases of certain diseases, of which Phthisis was one.

Under the direction of the local Sanitary Association, I was able to secure the willing help of about 30 contributors, and Returns of Phthisis, as well as of other diseases, were made with the greatest regularity for more than twelve years, and thus enabled the Medical Officer of Health to note any special incidence of the different diseases. They were also analysed by myself in Papers to the Social Science Congress, and to other kindred Societies.

There is good reason to believe that these "Weekly Returns" were not merely the forerunners but actual incentives to the more complete "Notification of Disease" that has been established in recent years.

Perhaps they may be counted as contributing to the storage of facts which led to the more active "Campaign," as also may my other works on Stethometry and Prognosis in Lung Diseases, but the first of the more militant Papers, a Health Lecture on "Foul Air and Lung Disease," was published by the Manchester and Salford Sanitary Association in 1876.

In the present Series, however, it has been thought best to commence with another Health Lecture, on "Consumption, its Causes and Prevention," as this lecture deals more directly with the subject.

It was not published until 1881, just before the discovery of the Tubercle bacillus, by Koch; but it contains nothing that runs counter to his research.

In this volume then are contained 22 Papers; and they are divided into 4 Sections. In each Section, they are placed in chronological order.

The Papers in the first Section are mainly practical in character; the second deals with the conditions of infection by Tubercle; the third contains original researches; and the Papers in the fourth are for the most part statistical in character.

Owing to the similarity of the subjects in these several series of Papers there is necessarily some repetition; but I have tried to minimise this defect as much as possible by omitting several Papers, especially those dealing with the conditions of infection.

Some little repetition may indeed be of service, as it may emphasise the doctrines which seem to me to be of most importance.

I wish here to express my gratitude to various kind friends who have helped me in preparing this volume; notably to Dr Dixon for the micro-photograph facing p. 172; to Mr G. Brumell, Dr Hope, Dr Newsholme and Dr Tatham for assistance with the Charts; and to Dr Venn and Mr J. W. Sharpe for correcting the proofs. Also my grateful acknowledgements of efficient assistance in my researches are due to Professor Delépine, the late Dr Dreschfeld, Drs Childs and Foulerton, and to Mr Harold Swithenbank.

A. R.

BOURNEMOUTH,
January 1915.

CONTENTS

LIST OF ILLUSTRATIONS

*available for download from www.cambridge.org/9781107418998

SECTION I. GENERAL

(1) CONSUMPTION: ITS CAUSES, AND ITS PREVENTION

HEALTH LECTURES FOR THE PEOPLE, *published by* **J**. *Heywood, for the Manchester and Salford Sanitary Association (Series 1881–82)*

IT has been thought well by the Committee of the Sanitary Association of this city that the subjects of its Health Lectures this year shall have reference to certain preventable diseases, and to the modes in which they may be prevented. The subject that has been assigned to me is a sufficiently sad one, and by many persons Consumption would be regarded as an inevitable evil— certainly not as one that can be averted by sanitary reforms. If this had been so, I hardly think I should have ventured to speak about it in an after-dinner discourse; but I trust that I shall prove that it is a distinctly preventable disease, and be able to show you how to prevent it.

There is no need for me to give you a medical description of this fell disease. It is so common, that I will venture to say that there is scarcely one amongst my hearers who has not had some one near and dear to him, a relative or a friend, affected by it. Most of you, then, know something of it, from its first insidious onset to its final painful ending—the loss of strength, the short hacking cough, the want of breath, the wasting of the flesh, the deceitful lulls in the course of the complaint, then the fever, the sweating, the distressing paroxysms of coughing and spitting, and, finally, the last scene of all, in which the overburdened spirit lays aside its worn-out garment of flesh.

R. 1

We know, too, the sad fact that most of the victims of this malady are the choicest specimens of our race. They are all carried off in the prime of manhood and womanhood, for the most part between the ages of 15 and 45. They are usually the flowers of the flock—the most intelligent, the most comely, the best and the bravest are singled out from our midst, and are often doomed to death before they have accomplished the tithe of the great things of which their talents had given such promise. They are cut down at the threshold of their career.

There is little need, then, to apologise for bringing before you a subject of so much importance—one that touches us all so nearly, and one that concerns, not individuals only, but the whole of the nation that is so heavily burdened by this disease. We are concerned now rather with the prevention of all this catalogue of evils, and the best way to understand them will be to try to find out their causes, and then how to remove them.

The first cause that must be mentioned is the obvious one of inheritance.

Everyone knows that `Consumption often runs in families. Some of you must have seen one member of a family after another struck down by this disease, and though this is sometimes capable of the explanation that the people all lived in the same locality, and in the same manner, yet there are many other instances of fathers and mothers being followed in this disease by sons and daughters, even though they have gone away from home and have altered entirely their mode of life. There are cases, too, in which the child is born with the disease already in its system. It is needless to say that here there can be no question of prevention, and if it were true that most cases of the disease are thus directly inherited, then, indeed, our task would be well-nigh a hopeless one, for very few families would then escape. Fortunately for our race, this is not so. It is an exceedingly rare event for a baby to be born with the seeds actually within its body.

What is meant by hereditary Consumption is very often nothing more than a weakness of constitution of such a nature that members of a consumptive family are more likely than others to take cold, and to get inflammation set up in their lungs, and then from these inflammations they make a very imperfect recovery—unhealthy inflammatory products are left in their systems, and then from these again true Consumption at last is developed.

Again, another way in which a consumptive tendency is inherited, is by means of an extreme sensitiveness to the peculiar poison, or the peculiar form of irritation, which provokes the disease, and this sensitiveness is often the greatest in the young. It is in this way that we can account for the fact of parents surviving their offspring. You may sometimes see the strange sight of a father and mother advanced in years, yet losing all their children one after another from Consumption. But you will generally find that when this is the case, the parents have come to their place of residence after their first youth, and that they had lived aforetime in some more healthy locality. They had got hardened, so to speak, before they came into the poison-laden atmosphere, and were able to resist its influence. The children, however, who came earlier in life within its grasp, were much less able to escape, and so they were carried off one by one.

You will easily see what a difference there is between the two latter forms of hereditary Consumption and the first. The two latter kinds are, in fact, not truly hereditary ; the patients have only inherited certain weaknesses of constitution, that render them prone to contract the malady. The positive lighting up of the Consumption depends upon external circumstances ; if these are not present, the disease will not become developed. Many of these circumstances are to a great extent, as we shall see presently, under our own control, and thus éven hereditary Consumption is, to a certain extent, a preventable disease.

The point is of the more importance, because, whilst directly transmitted Consumption is very rare, the two latter kinds of transmitted delicacy are very common, and may be dealt with by tens of thousands.

There are many persons, moreover—more than 60 per cent. of the whole number—in whom we can trace no hereditary taint, and yet they die of Consumption. Here, at any rate, there is little reason to doubt that it has been engrafted from without, and we may fairly ask, in the next place, what are the circumstances that are able to produce the disease in these people, and that will light it up still more readily in those who are disposed by constitution to take it.

It is natural to ask whether its prevalence has anything to do with climate. The disease is so common in England, and so many people leave our shores in the hope of finding some relief from it, that foreigners not unfrequently call it "the English disease"—and truly, it is very plentiful in this country. You have only to glance at the Table[1] to see that, in 10 years, in Manchester and Salford alone, a small army of 12,000 persons died of Consumption, and double this number of diseases of the lungs—more than a third of all the deaths; and in the same period, in England and Wales, more than half a million die of Consumption. It kills twice as many as any other disease. It is common enough here then; but it is by no means exclusively an English possession. It is just as bad in other countries (see the following table).

Proportion of Deaths from Consumption to 1000 *Deaths at*

London	121	Rome	114
Paris	143	Milan	132
Brussels	163	Lisbon	115
Vienna	208	Athens	183
Berlin	109	New York	167
Stockholm	160	Rio de Janeiro	186
Christiania	172	Lima	171
St Petersburg	151		(*Lombard.*)

If you compare the proportion of deaths from Consumption with the total deaths at the chief capital cities of the world, you will see that we are no worse, but generally better than our neighbours in this respect. It is in truth, as Dr Lombard calls it, "a ubiquitous malady"; it goes almost everywhere that man does; and it is worst where human beings are most crowded together. It is as bad or worse in the South as in the North, and in the East as in the West. In Europe, the only places comparatively free from it, are the sparsely peopled localities of Iceland, the Faroe Islands, the Hebrides of Scotland, the Highlands of Switzerland, and the almost desert steppes of the Wandering

---

[1] See Health Lecture on "Foul Air and Lung Disease," Heywood, Manchester and Salford Sanitary Association, 1878 (p. 63).

Tartars, or Kirghis. In Asia, although Persia is exempt, it is
common in India, and especially in Ceylon. In Pekin, it is the
chief cause of mortality. In the United States of America, it is
exceedingly prevalent, especially amongst women, and is increasing
in frequency; and in South America, in Brazil and in Valparaiso,
it is becoming every year more common. In many parts of the
vast space of Africa, as in the pure dry air of the upper Nile, for
instance, it is almost unknown; but it is beginning to be more
common along the coast, as it is also in the towns of Australasia.
In Algeria, it is remarked, and the remark is a very significant
one, that the free Arabs escape the disease entirely; but of the
captives, many die of Consumption. Assuredly, it has little or
nothing to do with climate.

The same truth is shown by the returns of the deaths from
Consumption in our army and navy, at the different stations to
which they are sent. You all know the proud boast that the sun
never sets upon the dominions of the Queen of England, and
wherever these are to be found our soldiers and sailors have to
go to look after and to protect them. Hence we get returns, and
exceedingly reliable ones, of the amount of mortality, and of the
diseases producing it, from all quarters of the globe. In the
annexed table this mortality is given at several stations for several
successive periods, and I think that you will be at once struck by
the enormous death rates amongst the troops in the earlier period,
and at every one of the stations.

Mortality per 1000 of Strength

	1830 to 1837	1837 to 1847	1863 to 1872	1874
Household Cavalry	14·5	11·1		
Cavalry of Line	15·3	13·5	9·17	8·79
Foot Guards	21·6	20·4		
Mediterranean Stations	21	16·4	11·2	7·27
Canada, etc.	23	17	9·49	6·0
Jamaica, etc.	91	59	17·05	16·9
Madras, India	52	—	24·22	14·22
Bengal, „	44			
Ceylon	49	—	21·95	6·04
Rates of Mortality at the same ages prevailing in healthy country populations				7·7
In England and Wales				9·2
In Manchester				12·4

In another diagram you have an opportunity of comparing this
mortality with that of the ordinary civil population of this country
at the same ages. You then see that the soldier died at three
times the rate of the civilian.

Again, on another diagram you may behold a representation of
what diseases it was that these soldiers principally died, and their
proportion to the same diseases in the ordinary civil population.
Both these diagrams refer, I am glad to say, to the earlier periods
of the history of the army, and you may see what cruel work
was wrought in its ranks by Consumption and by fevers of various
kinds. Here, then, again there is ample proof that Consumption
flourishes in all climates. But this table is valuable to us beyond
its purpose of proving the innocence of climate as a factor in the
production of Consumption. It is equally hard upon many of the
other theories of its causation, and, I may remark incidentally, it
shows that the causes are removable. It is an important witness
on the subject of inheritance. Dr Welch, of Netley, in his prize
essay on "Lung Disease Amongst Soldiers," tells us that, in the
army, cases of Consumption are not usually of the hereditary
form; and we can well understand that the doctors, who have to
examine recruits before they are allowed to pass into the ranks,
will take good care to accept those only who have a fairly clean
bill of health. Out of 1000 men thus examined at one time,
405 were rejected, and the minimum girth of the chest was
33 inches, a standard that is much above the civil average. The
requirements of height and of girth round the chest, and the
doctor's examination, ensure that the men shall be picked men and
in good health at the time of joining.

Other alleged causes of Consumption are equally excluded.
Thus it has been said that want of good nourishing food is a
cause. One of the latest writers on the subject[1] affirms that
the consumptive constitution is essentially "due to insufficient
nutrition, taking this word in its widest sense." And the same
statement is made by many English writers; but you all know
that the English soldier is always well fed, much better indeed
than the artizan and agricultural labourer, with whom we have
compared him, and who yet had three times the chance of life

[1] Dr Jaccoud, *Phthisie pulmonaire*, p. 7.

that he had. The same thing is proved by other facts. Thus
the ill-fed, ill-clothed fishermen of the Hebrides, exposed to all
vicissitudes of weather, hardly ever contract the disease ; but
the inhabitants of the mainland, though of the same race, die
at a high rate of Consumption ; and yet these are much better
fed, better clothed, and much better housed. We are told also
by Professor Hind that Consumption is unknown amongst the
natives of Labrador whilst they remain in their own country.
Here they live a kind of wild life in tents made of spruce branches,
imperfectly lined with skins, and more or less open on all sides to
the air. They are exposed to famine and all kinds of hardship ;
but when they come down the great river St Lawrence to take
part in the fisheries, they occupy well-built houses, and, being
well paid, they live in comparative luxury, and then many of
them, in the course of a year or two, become consumptive, and
thus miserably perish. From these facts we also gather that it
is not exposure to weather that will of itself produce the disease.
Nearly all the soldiers who died at the heavy rates here shown
lived in barracks, and were not on active service. Sailors, fishermen, sportsmen of all kinds, agricultural labourers, few of all
these are the victims of Consumption. No, but their better
protected neighbours in the towns · are ; and even their own
wives and daughters, who are obliged to keep the house, die at
twice or even three times the rate that they do themselves.

What, then, is the chief cause of all this frightful mortality
and misery ? What is there without which neither starvation,
exposure, nor hard work will bring on Consumption ? And, on
the other hand, what is there that is common to sick and poor—
that is to be found in all climates, in all collections of human beings,
and that is absent only in the places where Consumption is not to
be found—in two words, it is *foul air*. Think for a moment,
and you will see that this is true. The Royal Commission,
appointed after the Crimean War, to investigate the causes of
the excessive mortality of soldiers—this body of wise and careful
inquirers—came to the conclusion that the chief cause was the
faulty construction of barracks, especially in regard to ventilation
and to drainage. In England, the barracks were overcrowded
and badly ventilated and badly drained, and wherever the troops

were sent upon foreign service, there almost universally, except in India, where I may remark Consumption was least common, the same vicious mode of housing them was to be found. It is not surprising, then, that the Commission came to the conclusion that the heavy mortality, and especially the Consumption amongst soldiers, was due to the unhealthy barrack atmosphere. That they were correct is proved by the facts shown in the table, that sanitary reform in these respects at once altered the rate of mortality, and that, owing to the care which is now taken, it has become less than that of the ordinary working population of the country.

But there are several kinds of foul air, and there are also several kinds of Consumption. There is, moreover, some sort of relationship to be discovered between the two sets of events. It is notorious, for instance, that air filled with certain kinds of irritating dusts will provoke lung disease, ending, in many cases, in a form of Consumption. Thus the " dry grinders," as they are called, of Sheffield, suffered severely in this way, and so did the grinders of glass and earthenware, and the button-makers of Birmingham, and it is now proved conclusively that their lung diseases were due to irritating dust, for since the introduction of fans, that blow the dust away from the men's mouths, they have ceased to be so extensively punished by this complaint.

Even the catching of colds—the tendency to chronic bronchitis and asthma—maladies to which, as we have seen, people may have inherited a predisposition—even these have been shown to be due to a dusty, close, and foul atmosphere. But this brings us to another, and perhaps more important form of foul air, and to a form of Consumption that is still more common. By this kind of impurity, I mean the foulness that comes from the organic vapours that arise from the bodies of human beings. Our bodies are continually changing, from hour to hour, nay, from minute to minute. We take into them, in the course of a year, about a ton of food, and, in the course of the same time, the same amount of waste matter is got rid of. Now, a large part of this material is simply exhaled from our skins and from our lungs. It passes off in imperceptible flakes, or in the form of vapour. This it is that is the *chief* cause of Consumption. I do not say the only one (depressing conditions, want of exercise, stooping postures when at work, and other things have an influence), for that would be to overstate the case, but it is by far the most important and the most deadly. The proof of this statement, in order to be complete, would need to be established by a long string of evidence, such as I have no time now to detail to you, but it may be sufficient to say that it rests mainly upon the following facts :

1. Wherever people are collected together, the death rate from Consumption is in direct proportion to the degree of crowding together, and to the deficiency of ventilation. I will give only one instance of this, that was first remarked by Dr Guy—with reference to letter-press printers. He found that of 104 compositors who worked in rooms of less than 500 cubic feet for each person, 12·5 per cent. had had spitting of blood ; of 115 in rooms of from 500 to 600 cubic feet, 4·35 per cent. showed this sign of Consumption ; and in 100 who worked in rooms of more than 600 cubic feet capacity, less than 2 per cent. had spat blood. The direct relationship between crowding and Consumption is also well shown by the diagram on density of population and disease, from which you will see, at a glance, that Consumption increases as space diminishes.

2. In proportion as people are attracted to indoor occupations—and also in some degree in proportion to the solid impurities of the air—in such proportion do the various workpeople die of Consumption.

3. The theory explains the greater mortality from Consumption of the females in agricultural districts.

4. Animals exposed to impure air, or kept in close confinement, such as cows and monkeys, die of Consumption, just as human beings do—and when the direct experiment has been made of forcing rabbits and dogs to.inhale air, charged with filth of various kinds—especially the mucus from unhealthy lungs— they have at once become consumptive.

5. Lastly, in the light of these facts, we can readily explain the freedom from Consumption of the various places that I mentioned before. We saw that the Labrador fishermen lived in tents, with free access of air. The fishermen of the Hebrides live in huts, composed of stones loosely piled together, and the

reek from the peat, with which the interior is always filled, also probably possesses some power of destroying other noxious organic matter. In Persia, for six months of the year, the inhabitants sleep almost in the open air ; and in the cold season, in well ventilated houses. (*Lancereaux*.) In Switzerland, and in other high altitudes, the air for the most part is perfectly pure, and free from organic matter ; but even here there is no absolute freedom from the disease, when the air is allowed to become impure from the breath of many persons. Dr Emil Muller shows that the rate of mortality from lung disease—even in Switzerland—depends upon occupation. Industrial *indoor* pursuits give a rate varying from 10·2 to 4·7 per cent., and of these, one of the highest (9·8) is recorded at places of from 3400 to 4400 feet of altitude. In mixed labour, in districts at 4400 to 5000 feet of height, the rate is as high as 7·7 per cent.

In cold climates again, as of Iceland, Lapland, and Canada, we may probably ascribe the absence of Consumption to the purifying influence of frost. There is little doubt that the vapour of the air is the chief carrier of the peculiar poison that causes Consumption—and when this is condensed by the frost, it carries down with it much of the organic matter, and thus takes it out of the air of the room. The outer air also is thus purified to a very considerable extent.

The worst localities for Consumption are warm, damp, low situations, with impervious clay soils, and these also badly drained ; it will be readily seen that in those places there are no means of ridding the soil of animal impurities, and that the air over it is sure to be charged with moisture, and with vapours carrying with them the true seeds of Consumption.

There remains one other supposed cause of Consumption that I have not yet mentioned, and that is, fast living and intemperance. There is a popular impression abroad that this is a very common cause—but it has not yet been universally recognised amongst medical men. I am inclined to think myself that it is not a direct cause, but that it is a strong ally to other causes. It is certain that alcohol drinkers do suffer more from Consumption than total abstainers, in the proportion of six to four. Dr Dickinson, who made a special inquiry into the causes of the deaths of persons who trade in liquor, gives the above as the proportion, and he found that " Tubercle," as it is called, is twice as common in other organs than the lungs amongst those he terms the alcoholic class. And we need not be astonished at this result, for we know that the use of liquor renders men more liable to inflammation, and that this inflammation is not of a healthy kind, tending to repair, but rather to what is called degeneration.

We are now, I think, sufficiently prepared to consider the means by which Consumption may be prevented, and as I have stated its chief cause in two words, so the best means of preventing it may be summed up in three : (1) Ventilation, (2) Cleanliness, (3) Temperance, and these are placed in the order of their importance. They are applicable to all classes of the community.

You may, perhaps, have been surprised to find that I spoke of foul air as a cause common to rich and poor, and you may think that amongst the well-to-do the three preventive measures I have mentioned are fairly well attended to. But this is not so. As a general rule, the mansions of the rich are more completely closed up against the health-giving breezes of heaven than are the cottages of the poor, and though the windows of each room are, no doubt, opened for a certain time during the day, the refreshment that this gives lasts only for a very short time, and all the rest of the day the inhabitants of the rooms breathe an atmosphere that is full of danger to those who are predisposed to Consumption.

In the way of cleanliness again, no doubt the outside of the sepulchre is well whitened. There is the perfection of cleanliness about the living rooms, and even in the offices of the house. But what of the air ascending from the cellars ? Is not this often damp, and highly charged with organic matter, and is it not frequently the main source of continuous supply of so-called " fresh air " to the house ?

What revelations, too, have we not recently had as to the condition of the drainage of the better class of houses ? Owing to the very abundance of the various conveniences for cleanliness the modern mansion is often a mere receiver for sewer gas ; and in the more ancient family seat the attempts that have

been made to bring in modern luxuries have often succeeded in
introducing also the seeds of typhoid fever, diphtheria, or
dysentery, and, though last not least, the subtle sources of
tubercular disease.

Under the head of Temperance, we fortunately do not need
nowadays to inveigh against drunkenness amongst the upper
classes ; but there is still some fault to find in the injury to nutrition caused by intemperance in eating, by late hours, crowded
rooms, or a stifling atmosphere at theatres, balls, concerts, etc.
Few persons can realise how dangerous is even a temporary
exposure to such air, to those who are sensitive to the operation
of the poison.

Merchants and men of business and their clerks also often
inhabit close, stuffy offices during the day-time, and travel to
and from their work in crowded railway carriages or in fusty
omnibuses. I have often traced the origin of chest disease to
close confinement in the small ill-ventilated rooms that constitute
many of these places of business, where money may be made,
but where health is often lost.

Working men, as a rule, are in much less danger from their
daily employment. Although the atmosphere of workshops may
be full of irritating dusts of various kinds, and thus apt to
produce one form of lung disease, yet as a rule they are well
ventilated, and free from the pernicious organic foulness that is
so common a cause of true Consumption. Amongst working men
and their families it is in the evening and in the night that the
greater part of the mischief of this kind is done. In the crowded
clubrooms, or other worse places of entertainment, such as the
bar of a publichouse, but above all in the small bedrooms, often
far too full of occupants, and with doors and windows closely
shut to keep out the cold—often with the single outlet for foul
air, the chimney, stopped up with straw or a bundle of rags—
it is here that the worst forms of foul air are to be found,. and it
is in these places that Consumption is born and bred.

Let me then urge you all, and especially those who are predisposed to Consumption, to avoid a close atmosphere, both
night and day, as you would a deadly poison. Live regularly
and temperately, both as to eating and drinking ; and, lastly,

keep every part of your houses, every article of clothing, and the whole of the body, thoroughly clean. If you are also warmly clad, then, even in this climate, and in the smoky air of Manchester, you will almost certainly be able to ward off this fearful malady[1].

The subject of the cure of Consumption does not come within my present task; but I cannot let you go without expressing my own opinion, that in many cases the disease is quite curable, and that, for its cure, the same means that have been invoked for its prevention will be also powerful agents. In truth, the real reason why change of climate is so often ordered by medical men, and so often does good, is not because certain climates are particularly curative in themselves, but because invalids are thus often induced to be much out in the pure air.

It may perhaps be interesting to some, to state, in conclusion, that this is no new doctrine. Fresh air was enjoined by most of the great medical writers of olden time for the treatment of Consumption, or at any rate those things were enjoined that would best secure this ingredient. Hippocrates himself, in addition to a milk and fatty diet, enjoins exercise in the open air, such as a walk of from 10 to 15 miles daily. Aretæus prescribed milk and sea voyages; Celsus, a long sea voyage. Pliny speaks of the good influence of pine-woods, and of a diet containing the fat of goats, or plenty of milk and honey. Our great English physician, Sydenham, ordered horse exercise, and a milk diet; and he is followed in this by Van Swieten and others. And I may sum up all these doctrines very well in an old doggerel rhyme that was published in the last century:

> " If Consumption cured can be,
> Which is a mighty rarity;
> These three things you must prepare,
> Milk, traumatics[2], and fresh air."

---

[1] As to the means to be taken to secure the above requisites, I must refer to the Health Lectures of previous years, which enter into details on all these points.

[2] Blisters or issues.

(2) ON THE PREVENTION OF CONSUMPTION

Lecture to Congress, September 22, 1887

WHEN I was asked to deliver a lecture before the Sanitary Congress at Bolton, I felt some little hesitation in bringing before it the subject of the Prevention of Consumption.

The prevention of disease is indeed the aim of all sanitary reformers, and I had little doubt as to the acceptability of an address aiming, with any likelihood of success, at the prevention of a disease of such importance as consumption.

But this was just the point at which some misgiving would creep in, and the question would arise as to whether there was sufficient evidence of the preventability of tubercular disease, as to justify me in bringing the subject before the members of this great Institute.

I think there is, but before venturing to bring my views before this meeting, I thought it well to ask for the permission of your council.

This permission has now been freely given to me, and I must therefore proceed to defend my thesis as well as I am able—and to lay before you the reasons for my faith, and my grounds for thinking that this fell disease, the " scourge of England " as it has been called, may reasonably be called preventable, and by what means it may be prevented or at least be limited in its range.

I need not dilate much upon the magnitude of the task before us. About 70,000 persons die every year of tubercular disease in England and Wales, and as the average duration of the disease is now about three years, this means that there are nearly 200,000 persons in the country constantly suffering from the complaint.

How fatal consumption is to the adult part of the population, may be judged from the fact that more than a quarter of the total deaths between the ages 15 and 65 are caused by it, and nearly half between 15 and 35.

> " To see it down in figures on a page,
> Plain, silent, clear, as 'God sees through the earth
> The sense of all the graves, that's terrible
> For one who is not God, and cannot right
> The wrong he looks on."   *Aurora Leigh.*

It is the working years of men's lives that are chiefly affected by consumption. It is the malady of youth and middle life, and thus interferes more than any other with the economy of the State.

It carries off the most efficient of the population in the prime of manhood or of womanhood, and many of them are those who have given bright promises for the future.

Consumption often carries off the flower of the flock—the most intelligent, the comeliest, the bravest and the best. They are cut down before they have accomplished a tithe of the great things of which their talents have given promise. Few can have failed to notice that many of those promising young people who have been thought worthy of biographical fame have finally succumbed to the onset of this fell malady.

The very magnitude of the work before us, and its extreme importance, is indeed the best excuse that I can give for bringing it before you ; and if it can be proved to be within the bounds of possibility that such a disease can be prevented, the greatness of the task ought surely to be an additional incentive to attempt it, according to the Latin saying, " dignus vindice nodus."

But, up to quite a recent period, not only was consumption deemed to be incurable, it was also regarded as almost inevitable. Families in which existed the taint of the disease were supposed to be doomed : a certain number of them were certain to succumb to the hereditary curse.

Insurance offices still refuse to enrol amongst their members those who have lost father and mother from the disease, and even collateral relatives who have died from it are judged to have an influence upon the life of the candidate for life assurance.

It was also common amongst workpeople who worked at unhealthy trades, such as steel-grinding, glass-cutting, mining, etc., to regard the mortality from consumption amongst them as only natural and part of their fate. A fork-grinder once said to Mr Hall, of Sheffield, " I shall be thirty-six next month, and you know that is getting an old man at our trade." And another, a young man of about twenty-six years, said he " reckoned in about two more years at his trade he might begin to think of dropping off the perch " ; adding, " You know a knife-grinder is an old cock at thirty."

Whilst these forebodings were held with regard to those who came of a consumptive stock, and those who followed certain trades, the fate of the consumptive himself was regarded as hopeless.

In my student days I have over and over again seen physicians regard the stethoscopic sounds that revealed the commencement of tubercle as equivalent to a sentence of death, and even the late Sir Thomas Watson, in his classical work on the *Practice of Physic*[1], says : " The tubercular disease when established is beyond our power."

Niemeyer again remarks : " Many a patient gets well, who would formerly have been assumed to be a victim of tubercular and therefore incurable disease. I am fully convinced from my own experience of the last few years that in former times I lost many a patient from galloping consumption, only because I considered him lost from the very first[2]."

Even before the discovery of the bacillus of tubercle, these views of the inevitable character and the incurability of consumption were already beginning to be doubted.

It was shown by Dr Pollock, in his work on the *Elements of Prognosis in Consumption*[3], that : " Many cases which were given up by doctors, but outlived the prediction to arrive at old age, were undoubtedly recoveries from phthisis. Many more were instances of an early invasion of the disease with subsidence of the symptoms and long tolerance of the deposit." Again, he says : " I have many times witnessed all the phenomena of deposit,

[1] Vol. II. p. 201.   [2] *Lecture on Consumption*, p. 65.
[3] p. 68.

and all the symptoms of phthisis entirely removed[1]." " The best
authorities lean to the opinion that tubercle is capable of removal
by absorption[2]."

Dr T. C. Williams remarks that the animal matter of tubercle
may be absorbed ; and Dr Carswell says, " the curability of this
disease has in my opinion been settled by Laennec " ; and my
old master, Dr Stokes of Dublin, says, " there is no doubt that
modern practice has proved the curability of phthisis," adding,
" it is probable that many more cases of phthisis recover than is
supposed[3]."

I have myself seen many cases of what might fairly be called
cure, seeing that the patients lived thirty or forty years after
undoubted cavities had formed in their lungs. Still more frequently have I recorded cases in which incipient disease had been
arrested, and no physical signs were to be found afterwards in the
lungs. Within the last twenty years also it has become evident
that there has been a distinct diminution in the death-rate from
phthisis throughout the country.

In the three years, 1858 to 1860, the annual rate of mortality
from consumption per million of persons living was 2567. In
1884 it was only 1818, a diminution of 749 per million, or a total
saving of about 20,000 lives every year.

Nor is this improvement confined to England. "In 1857,
39·50 deaths from consumption were returned in the State of
Massachusetts for each 10,000 of the population ; in 1883 only
29·90. This decrease is too large to credit to greater accuracy in
diagnosis and to the transference of consumption to other States,
and is mainly attributable to the prevention of phthisis by improved hygiene[4]."

Evidence has also been forthcoming of the strongest kind, of
the influence of sanitary measures, and especially of good drainage
and good ventilation, as a preventative of consumption.

No better instance of this could be found than in the records
of the mortality from this disease in the British army and navy.
This evidence was collected by the Commission on the Sanitary State
of the Army in 1858; and the results are shown in the following

[1] p. 117.   [2] p. 119.   [3] Lectures in 1835.
[4] Strumpel, *Text Book of Medicine*, p. 213.

table which has frequently been quoted before, but which can hardly be too often brought before public notice. This mortality is given at several stations for several successive periods, and I think that you will be at once struck by the enormous death-rates amongst the troops in the earlier period, and at every one of the stations, and by the great reduction of the rate in 1874. At the present time it is still further reduced[1].

Mortality per 1000 *of Strength.*

	1830 to 1837	1837 to 1847	1863 to 1872	1874
Household Cavalry	14·5	11·1		
Cavalry of Line	15·3	13·5	9·17	8·79
Foot Guards	21·6	20·4		
Mediterranean Stations	21	16·4	11·2	7·27
Canada, etc.	23	17	9·49	6·0
Jamaica, etc.	91	59	17·05	16·9
Madras, India	52		24·2	14·22
Bengal „	44	—		
Ceylon....................	49	—	21·95	6·04

Rates of Mortality at the same ages prevailing in healthy country populations ..	..	..	..	..	..	7·7
In England and Wales	..	..	..	..	..	9·2
In Manchester	..	..	..	..	..	12·4

The greater part of this excessive mortality was due to consumption.

Dr Buchanan, now medical officer to the Local Government Board, has also conclusively shown that good drainage of a locality may diminish by one half the prevalence of the disease, as in the case of the city of Salisbury.

These proofs of the preventability of consumption were accumulated long before the discovery by Prof. Koch, that in most cases the disease originates outside the body, that it is due to the minute micro-organism named by him the bacillus of tubercle, and that its ravages are fostered by various external conditions, most of which are undoubtedly under the control of appropriate sanitary measures.

---

[1] In 1883 it was only 6·28 per 1000, and throughout the world only 9·57.

Since then it has become increasingly evident that Louis was right when he said, that " few persons were born necessarily to die of the disease," and it has been now abundantly proved that consumption is eminently a preventable disease.

But before proceeding at once to the inquiry how it may be prevented, let us for a few moments consider what tubercle is now ascertained to be. An amusing imaginary conversation, given by Dr McCormack, will serve to show the stride that has been recently made in our knowledge on this point.

" If you ask a pathologist what tubercle is, he will perchance reply, readily, that it is a certain deep-seated or, peradventure, superficial tumour which possibly tends to suppuration. You quietly remind him, that you do not ask where it is seated or to what it proceeds, but only what it really is. He will then, it may be, inform you that there are tubercles yellow, gray, and miliary, nay fibroid, induced by depressed vital powers, in short a defective decaying tendency in the bioplasm. You rejoin as gently as may be, that you do not care a button about their colour or size, and as for depressed vital powers you consider that mere φλυαρία, since you only desire to learn what tubercles actually are.

" The pathologist now takes himself up a little, as a Frenchman might say, and briskly states that tubercle in fact is a morbid material which, being deposited on the mucous and serous surfaces and in the areolar tissues, destroys the elements which it implicates. In the excess of your courtesy you beg his pardon, and just remark that you do not want to learn where the material in question is deposited or what tissue it destroys, but only what it assuredly is. By this time our pathologist's colour becomes ever so little heightened ; still he answers confidently that tubercle, as resulting from a pathological alteration, degenerates into an opaque, then a friable, lastly a purulent substance, which—. But here you boldly interrupt him with the observation that not yet has he replied to your inquiry as to the real nature and essence of tubercle. The pathologist, if he be a candid person, as pathologists commonly are, then confesses, as he might just as well have done at the outset, that he knows nothing whatever, the real nature of tubercle regarded, about the matter."

Fortunately we know something more than this now of the

intimate nature of tubercle. Thanks to Prof. Koch we know that it is constantly associated with the presence of a micro-organism which, either by its own initiative power, or by means of the products of its activity, causes the formation of the bodies called tubercles within the textures of the body ; that it makes its entrance from without ; and that, once lodged within the frame, it travels infectively through it, chiefly along the course of the lymphatic system.

The conditions of its existence are briefly those to be found within the animal body—a certain degree of moisture, a temperature of about 37° Centigrade (from 86° to 107° F.), and a supply of nitrogenous food, such as blood serum will give.

If cultivated outside the body all these conditions must be imitated, and there is further the very important observation that it needs for its development a sojourn of at least a week, and sometimes much longer, in these conditions before it can take root, so to speak, and grow. Moreover, it is a being of very tenacious vitality, and it will preserve its virulence and capacity for development for six weeks or longer in decomposing tuberculous material, and for six months at least in a dry state. It also resists the action of many germicides.

Its close connection with tubercle has been proved, (1) by its almost constant presence in tuberculous cases ; (2) by its absence in all other diseases ; and (3) by pure cultivations of its colonies, injected into the body, causing tubercular disease of the parts inoculated.

Once in the body, there is unfortunately hardly a structure which tubercle does not implicate, or a function which primarily or secondarily in its sequences it does not invade and derange. As Dr McCormack forcibly says, " No tongue could narrate, no pen indeed declare, its deplorably frightful ravages. The exquisitely beautiful fabric of the eye does not escape, much less, with all their admirable mutual adjustments, the muscles, joints, and bones. The entire living material fabric, this so magnificent handiwork of God, is in truth disintegrated, defaced, and destroyed. The interior and exterior tissues waste and wither, the fingers become misshapen, the nails curve over, the muscles both of organic life and the life of relation, no longer adequately nourished, lose their volume, the lung tissue, as Rokitansky tells us, ulcerates and disappears. The breath is as if from a vault, and in laryngeal phthisis, the poor sufferer, spitting, choking, coughing, is perhaps carried off by suffocative spasm of the glottis at last."

Now, how may consumption be prevented? The answer to this question depends upon the reply to the further inquiry—what are the conditions that enable the tubercle bacillus to enter the body in a virulent form, and what further are those that enable it to do its deadly work there? As Cicero has aptly said, "Physicians consider that, when the cause of a disease has been discovered, they have also discovered its cure." At least if this is not quite true they can often prevent it.

Let us first dispose of a number of influences, formerly supposed to be causes of consumption, that have now been proved to have only a remote or doubtful effect upon its course.

1. *Climate.* At one time it was supposed that climate was everything, both in the prevention and cure of consumption, but it has now been shown to be almost entirely without influence, except so far as it permits or discourages an almost entirely open air life.

Wherever human beings are congregated together, in every part of the habitable globe, and in all climates, there is consumption to be found. It is, as Dr Lombard says, "a ubiquitous malady."

It would almost be sufficient to point to the table of Army Mortality for the proof of this assertion, but I have also drawn up a table from Dr Lombard's statistics showing its great prevalence in most of the capital cities of Europe, and in other parts of the world (p. 4).

It will be seen that it is almost as prevalent in the South as in the North, in the East as in the West.

Even in the places where there is the greatest exemption from the disease, as in the desert, on high mountain ranges, and in Arctic or Sub-Arctic regions, it is still to be found under certain unsanitary conditions. In Asia Minor it is often met with on the coast and in the principal towns. The Bedouins on the coast of the Red Sea, "who exchange their tents for stone-built houses," suffer from it. In Syria it is met with at Aleppo, and in the Soudan at Khartoum.

In Algeria whilst the nomad Arabs are free, "amongst the captives many die of the disease."

The same observations may be made regarding Australia and North and South America, including Canada and the Arctic regions.

Even in the high lands of Switzerland there is no complete immunity from the disease. Amongst those of the population who are attracted to indoor employments, as Dr Emil Müller has shown[1], a certain proportion die of the disease. Industrial indoor pursuits give rise to a rate varying from 6·5 to 10·2 per cent., and one of the highest of these rates, 9·8, is at an elevation of 3400 to 4400 feet. At 4400 to 5000 feet of altitude, in mixed labour the rate from the disease was 7·7 per cent.

Here, then, again we find the conditions of life a much more powerful influence than climate or elevation of site.

2. Take next exposure to cold, privation, and hardship of all kinds ; only remotely are these causes of consumption.

It is true that there are still medical men who regard them as the chief agents in preparing the human frame for its ravages ; thus Dr Jaccoud affirms that the consumptive constitution is essentially due to "insufficient nutrition, taking this word in its widest sense," and Mon. Bouchardat, in his recent treatise on Hygiene, affirms that "the continuous loss of calorific elements, in any considerable proportion, leads to pulmonary tuberculosis," and that it is due to some form of "misère physiologique."

But the Army Medical Reports again afford a sufficient answer to this hypothesis. The phthisis that at one time carried off so many of the finest soldiers of the British army, was not brought on by starvation, or privation, or exposure to hardship. It occurred for the most part when they were not on active service, but in the time of peace, when they were well fed and well cared for in every material respect, far better in fact than the half-starved artisans and agricultural labourers, who died at only one-third the rate that they did.

Again, the poor fishermen of Iceland, and the hunters and trappers of North America, the nomad tribes of Asia and Africa,

[1] *Distribution of Consumption in Switzerland.*

the wretched natives of Australia, all these people escape the disease almost entirely, whilst half the deaths of the well-protected, well-clothed, adult inhabitants of towns, are from this cause.

The Highlanders who inhabit well-built houses on the mainland of Scotland are subject to the same rate as the other inhabitants; whilst the ill-fed, ill-clothed fishermen of the Hebrides, who are of the same race, hardly ever contract the disease.

It is quite true that inflammations of the respiratory apparatus, especially of the tissues of the lungs and pleura, constitute a remote or predisposing cause of consumption. These diseases are apt to destroy the natural elasticity of the lungs, and render them unable to dislodge or to destroy the micro-organism which may succeed in finding an entrance into them, and which thus may plant itself firmly into their substance, irritating them and ultimately leading to consolidation and subsequent softening.

If the conditions are such as to lead people easily to take cold, and if they thus produce what is called chronic catarrhal pneumonia, they leave a condition of the lungs that both facilitates the lodgment in them of the tubercle bacillus, and also prevents its expulsion or destruction by the natural forces of the human economy. Some physicians believe that nearly all cases of phthisis commence in this way. Niemeyer says, " Tuberculosis is in most cases a secondary disease " ; and Dr Herman Weber observes, " A fruitful source of phthisis is the tendency to catarrh of the respiratory mucous membrane " ; and he further points out how these catarrhs may lead to phthisis : " (1) By producing numerous mucous abrasions upon which the bacilli can settle ; (2) by weakening epithelial cells and their ciliary action ; (3) by rendering respirations more shallow ; and (4) by weakening the nutrition and energy of the whole system."

In the light of modern research it is not difficult to understand why a loss of elasticity of the lung should lead to consumption. We have seen that the bacillus of tubercle needs for its development a sojourn of at least a week in contact with suitable nourishment, and at a temperature nearly approximating to that of the human body. It is also highly probable that in all towns and wherever men most congregate some of these infective particles are present in the atmosphere, but they are for the most part quite harmless to healthy persons. One reason why they are thus harmless may well be the difficulty with which these particles make their way along the air passages of the lungs of such people. They are constantly liable to be arrested on the moist surfaces of the mucous membrane ; and, if they are once caught in this way, they will soon be passed out of the chest by the delicate " cilia " that line the tubes. Even if they should penetrate into the ultimate lung tissues also, they are likely to be destroyed by the fresh blasts of air that rush freely into every portion of a healthy lung.

These safeguards, however, are not present in lungs that have either been compressed by constrained postures, or that have lost their elasticity through inflammatory actions. The germs of the disease, therefore, if they can penetrate the inactive portions of such damaged lungs, may find there both suitable food and warmth, and may rest long enough to develope true tubercular irritation.

In complaints such as simple catarrh and bronchitis, in which there is a copious secretion of mucus, I am inclined to think that there is less reason to fear a permanent lodgment of the bacillus. This organism is, in fact, likely to be entangled in the frothy secretion, and to be expelled along with it before it can do harm.

Some years ago, in an inquiry into the nature and quantity of the organic matter of the breath, I was much struck with the fact that in bronchitis and catarrh, and other diseases in which there was much expectoration, the proportionate amount of this substance exhaled in the aqueous vapour from the lungs was only one half of that from healthy persons ; not that there was really less organic matter thus excreted, but because it was taken up by the mucus before it could reach the mouth.

Professor Tyndall has also shown, by means of his illuminated tube, " the filtering action " of the lungs—all dust inhaled being caught up by the bronchial secretion and prevented from appearing in the expired air. It would equally be prevented from travelling into the air cells. Something of this kind must always go on in such diseases as those in question.

But even in chronic bronchitis, after a time, the expulsive machinery may become defective, the waving cilia may become less active, the muscular apparatus of the tubes may be weakened, and dilatation and plugging of the air passages may occur ; thus the bacillus may find a lodgment within the lungs, and true tubercular disease may be set up. This specific infection is again still more likely to take place if from any cause the ultimate tissues become inflamed, as in the various forms of catarrhal-pneumonia or broncho-pneumonia. In this case, even more than in simple catarrh, the lung loses its elasticity, its tissues are more open to infection, the residual air becomes stagnant, and its impurities, including foreign germs, are liable to be imprisoned for an indefinite time. In such a sense as this then, the causes of inflammatory diseases of the chest are also the causes of consumption.

But is exposure to the elements as fruitful a cause of cold-catching as is commonly supposed ? Do we find that men who are much in the open air are more likely to take cold than the inmates of well warmed and well closed apartments ? Quite the contrary. Soldiers on campaign, sailors, fishermen, hunters, gipsies, engine-drivers, coachmen, gardeners, agricultural labourers, none of these people suffer much from catarrhal affections, unless they are intemperate. To quote again from Dr McCormack[1], " Arctic explorers, supplied indeed with food and clothes, confront with perfect equanimity the chilliest air that ever flowed. Whymper safely slept, he tells us, *sub divo*, in chill Alaska, with only a screen to windward, when the mercury in his barometer was frozen hard. Von Wrangel relates quite a similar experience in respect of the dwellers by the shores of the Arctic ocean."

It is interesting to notice also the immunity from cold exhibited by our volunteers when they camp out for a week or a fortnight, and the instance has the more value because most of these men are unaccustomed to an open air life, and have for the most part of their days been the occupants of close offices or stuffy warehouses.

I have known men to be thus exposed for a great part of their time not only to cold, but to drenching rain, with pools forming under their beds in the tents, and yet not a single man in a battalion has been invalided from the effects of cold.

On the other hand we know that the inhabitants of towns not

[1] p. 40.

only contract diseases of the lungs, but die of their consequences in excessive numbers. It has been calculated that in Manchester people die of these complaints at more than three times the rate that they do in breezy Westmoreland. Mere exposure to cold, and hardship, and privation, is not therefore to be reckoned as a cause of consumption.

3. The next supposed cause of consumption to which I shall allude is the inhalation of irritating substances, or dusts, arising from works of various kinds, such as steel grinding, glass cutting, brush making, etc.

In the year 1858, Dr Headlam Greenhow presented to the Privy Council a report in which he pointed out the influence of occupation as a cause of pulmonary diseases. In 1860 and 1861, he returned again to the subject, and dwelt especially upon the large mortality from these complaints amongst those who worked in an atmosphere impregnated with dust consisting of fine particles of metal or of sandstone, etc.

His statistics, although very valuable in many ways, are nevertheless open to criticism in reference to the causation of consumption. He groups together many very different forms of lung affection—many that are not tuberculosis at all—and he was not able in many cases to discriminate between the effects of the occupation itself, and those of the conditions under which it was carried on.

No one, indeed, who has studied the vital statistics of these occupations, or who has medically attended the workpeople, can doubt the power of irritating dusts in inducing a state of the lungs that is favourable to the reception of the specific organism.

Just as in the case of lungs otherwise injured, tubercle may readily be engrafted upon a miner's or a needlemaker's lung ; but the disease that is first caused by the particles these men inhale is not tuberculous at all. It is simply a chronic inflammation, affecting chiefly the connective tissue and causing the formation of a fibroid tissue in the alveolar walls. It leads ultimately to a contraction, and, so to speak, a strangling of certain portions of the lung tissue. But no bacilli are found either in the tissues or in the expectoration of such patients, as I can testify from frequent stainings.

I have myself watched many of these cases, occurring in persons who have lived under otherwise healthy conditions; and although they have ultimately succumbed to the exhausting effects of the disease, yet from first to last they have kept free from the infection of tubercle. The cirrhosis, or fibroid disease, as it has been called, never degenerated into true consumption.

Dusts, therefore, although they are a serious danger, and though they ought on this account to be kept away from work-people, as a preventive measure against consumption, are yet only remotely a cause of the disease. Much the same must be said of stooping postures during work.

4. I would say a few more words on the subject of hereditary predisposition to the disease.

That this is a real source of danger no medical man would deny. Thus we have seen instances of families in which almost every member has died of the disease, and others in which members of the same family, living in different and far distant places, have yet one and all ultimately succumbed to it. In every such instance however, so far as I am aware, something has been added to the mere vulnerability of the persons attacked, either residence in confined air, repeated attacks of cold or some other assisting cause. And such a tendency to contract the disease can only be regarded as a remote and not as an essential cause of consumption. There is no need to assume the existence of a tubercular consti-tution any more than there is for affirming that there is a diph-theritic or typhoid constitution, when a family is unusually pre-disposed to any of these disorders.

I know, for instance, of one family in which six out of eleven children have died of diphtheria, and other members have suffered from the complaint. They were not all struck down at the same time nor by the same epidemic; but three children died in one place, one at another, and two in the village where they are now residing. Such a fatality as this from a particular disease means nothing more than a tendency to contract it, and a readiness to give way before its attacks.

It is, moreover, highly probable that heredity has much less to do with consumption than is commonly supposed. A very large proportion of cases arise without any phthisical family history in the past. Many healthy families leaving the country and coming to reside in crowded towns subsequently lose some members from consumption. In the army more than 60 per cent. of cases are non-hereditary. Even when we take the difficult test of statistics, we find they are apt to be deceptive. Thus Briquet found that one-third of the consumptive patients at a hospital were born of consumptive parents on one side or the other ; Dr Quain, 25 per cent. ; Dr T. C. Williams, 12 per cent. of direct influence, and 48 per cent. of family predisposition. But in these figures no account is taken of the influence of external circumstances, circumstances that are common to all the members of the family.

Again, there are so many deaths from phthisis in this country (as I said before, about half of all the deaths between the ages of 15 and 35 are due to this cause), that, without any such thing as hereditary taint, there would be nothing surprising in the fact that half of the consumptive patients have had consumptive relatives.

Dr Walshe, the chief authority on chest diseases in this country, obtained from his hospital patients the result that about 26 per cent. came of a father or mother, or of both parents, similarly diseased ; but, in discussing the significance of these figures, he asks whether they prove the reality of hereditary influence, and decides that they do not. " This ratio," he says, " of 26 per cent. might be, and probably is, no higher than that of the tuberculized portion of the population generally," and he concludes that " much phthisis is, in each generation, non-hereditary."

In any case it is highly probable that this influence has been greatly overrated. If the true causes of consumption are avoided, even those who come of a consumptive stock will escape the hereditary curse. As Louis says[1] : " Nous n'avons recueilli aucun fait en faveur de l'hérédité de la phthisie."

We are now prepared to consider certain conditions that seem to be more essential than others to the virulent activity of the micro-organism.

The Commission on the Sanitary State of the Army in 1858, whose report I have already quoted, recognised as chief agents two causes, and affirmed plainly that " the ravages committed in the

[1] *Recherches sur la Phthisie*, p. 532.

ranks of the army by pulmonary disease are to be traced in a great degree to the vitiated atmosphere generated by overcrowding and deficient ventilation, and *the absence of proper sewerage of barracks*. In 1864 Mr A. B. Middleton also called attention to these two sources of danger in a paper read before the British Association at Bath ; but in an independent inquiry conducted in 1862 in Massachusetts by Dr Bowditch, the extreme importance of dampness of soil as a cause of consumption was insisted upon.

He came to the conclusion that—(1) " A residence on or near a damp soil, whether that dampness is inherent in the soil itself or caused by percolation from adjacent ponds, from marshes, or springy soils, is one of the primal causes of consumption in Massachusetts, probably in New England, and possibly in other portions of the globe. (2) Consumption can be checked in its career, and possibly, nay probably, prevented by attention to this law."

Shortly afterwards, and without any knowledge of Dr Bowditch's conclusions, Dr Buchanan, who is now the chief medical officer to the Local Government Board, came to much the same conclusions as the result of an elaborate research into the distribution of consumption in the three south-eastern counties of England beyond the limits of the Metropolis.

His conclusions are well worthy of being quoted *in extenso*. They are as follows :

(1) Within the counties of Surrey, Kent, and Sussex, there is, broadly speaking, less phthisis (*i.e.* consumption) among populations living on pervious soils than among populations living on impervious soils.

(2) Within the same counties there is less phthisis among populations living on high-lying pervious soils than among populations living on low-lying pervious soils.

(3) Within the same counties there is less phthisis among populations living on sloping impervious soils than among populations living on flat impervious soils.

(4) The connection between soil and phthisis has been established in this inquiry—(*a*) by the existence of general agreement in phthisis mortality between districts that have common geological and topographical features of a nature to affect the

water-holding quality of the soil ; (*b*) by the existence of general disagreement between districts that are differently circumstanced in regard to such features; and (*c*) by the discovery of pretty regular concomitancy in the fluctuation of the two conditions, from much phthisis with much wetness of soil, to little phthisis with little wetness of soil. But the connection between wet soil and phthisis came out last year in another way, which must here be recalled— (*d*) by the observation that phthisis had been greatly reduced in towns where the water of the soil had been artificially removed, and that it had not been reduced in other towns where the soil had not been dried.

(5) The whole of the foregoing conclusions combine into one —which may now be affirmed generally, and not only of particular districts—that " wetness of soil is a cause of phthisis to the population living upon it."

(6) No other circumstance can be detected, after careful consideration of the materials accumulated during this year, that coincides on any large scale with the greater or less prevalence of phthisis, except the one condition of soil.

These results have since been confirmed by Dr Haviland, and by the Registrar General of Scotland. In the conclusions drawn from his map of the distribution of phthisis in England and Wales, Dr Haviland says : " Damp, clayey soil, whether belonging to the wealden, oolitic, or cretaceous formation, is coincident with a high mortality " ; and the Registrar General, in his seventh report, remarks that " the towns, villages, hamlets, or houses, which are situated at or near undrained localities, or are on heavy, impermeable soils, or on low-lying ground, and whose sites are consequently kept damp, had a very much larger number and proportion of cases of consumption than towns, villages, hamlets, or houses which are situated on dry or rocky ground, or on light porous soils, where the redundant moisture easily escapes."

The vapours that arise from damp ground, and which make their way into houses, are often very impure and charged with organic matter that may be a suitable food for the tubercle bacillus.

In an address to this Congress, held at Leicester, the year before last, I gave the details of an inquiry into this subject that goes even further than those already cited—a contrast between two populations, one being resident on clay lands, the other on a hill of sand. The result was derived from a ten years mortality table, and was that whereas in this period there had originated forty-four cases per 1000 inhabitants on the clay lands, on the sand only one per 1000 had thus suffered, and that not one of the children or females of the population who were constantly resident there had contracted the disease. In this instance, however, we had only the influence of a dry soil to deal with ; the houses were those of well-to-do people, and were fairly well ventilated. Whether there would have been the same immunity under other conditions is very doubtful.

Still it is evident from the facts before us that there is a close relationship between the condition of the soil and consumption— a relationship so close that, as we have seen, a residence on a porous soil, under otherwise favourable hygienic conditions, will apparently preserve the whole community from the disease.

It is further noticeable that in these cases hereditary predisposition made no difference in the result. There were present in these populations many whose parents or near relatives had died of the disease, and yet they did not contract it so long as they lived in the place. I think it may therefore be fairly assumed that in a well-drained, uncontaminated soil, we have one of the means by which consumption may be prevented.

But we still have to consider the most prolific source from which the bacillus of tubercle derives its virulence—a cause without which neither starvation, nor exposure, nor hard work, not even probably hereditary predisposition, will bring on consumption. It is a cause that is common to rich and poor, that is to be found in all climates, in all collections of human beings, and that is only absent in the places where consumption is not to be found. In two words, it is *foul air*, and for the most part it is air that has been rendered foul by previous respiration.

It is to Dr McCormack that we owe the most definite statement of this now well-recognised influence, that, as he says, there " wherever there is foul air...there we meet consumption, we meet scrofula, and an untimely death."

His further theory that tubercle is due to " carbon and other impurities inadequately discharged during the process of respiration " is now not tenable, but his demonstration of the danger of breathing air that has been breathed before is of none the less value.

Let me very briefly bring before you the grounds for this opinion :

1. We have the fact that increased density of a population means also increased general mortality, and especially increased mortality from lung disease. The late Dr Farr was the first to establish this fact, and to reduce it almost to a mathematical demonstration.

In proportion as larger and larger numbers of persons are attracted to a certain limited area of ground, in that proportion, *caeteris paribus*, does the mortality from consumption increase.

It is true that we have along with this condition a combination of most, if not all, of the other circumstances unfavourable to health—poverty, insufficient food, low site and often damp ill-constructed dwellings ; and we might with equal right select any one of these things as the true cause of the disease, but for the fact that all these things exist, in still greater intensity, in some country districts of England, or in the poorer villages of Scotland, along with a very low rate of mortality from consumption.

2. We have the evidence, that is now most ample, that in proportion as people are attracted to indoor occupation, and in proportion to the degree of closeness and bad ventilation of the places in which they work, in that proportion is the rate of mortality from consumption increased. This fact was first demonstrated by Dr Greenhow in his statistical inquiry, but it has since been fully confirmed by other observers.

Any one who looks at the map of the distribution of consumption in England, prepared by Mr Alfred Haviland, must be at once struck with the deepening of colour that shows intensity of disease in the great industrial centres of the country. The influence of this cause is also shown by the contrast between the male and female rates of mortality in town and country districts.

In some parts of England the men are the chief workers at indoor employments—as in Sheffield and Birmingham ; there you find the male rate the highest ; in others, as at Nottingham, Huddersfield, and Macclesfield, the women are most employed, and consequently they die most numerously of consumption ; and in places like Liverpool, Manchester, and Stockport, where there is little difference in the employment of men and women, there is also little difference in the rates of mortality from consumption ; both are high.

But the most striking testimony is from the relative death-rates in the two sexes in country places, such as Market Drayton, Bakewell, Nuneaton, Camelford, and Pickering. Here, where the men are constantly out of doors, their consumption rate is uniformly low, while the women, who keep the house, die at a constantly higher rate of this disease. (See also Table III, p. 104).

3. We have the experience given to us by the records of the mortality from consumption in the British Army and Navy, and a similar history could be told of the other European forces.

In the exhaustive report of the Commission upon the Sanitary State of the Army, it appeared that lung disease was more than twice as fatal amongst the picked men who formed the army as it was amongst the ordinary civil population of the country (12·5 of the former to 5·8 of the latter).

They pointed out that in civil life, insufficient clothing, insufficient and unwholesome food, sedentary and unwholesome occupations, and the vitiated atmosphere of unhealthy dwellings, all contribute to the propagation of this class of diseases. But in the army it cannot be alleged that the clothing, the food, or the nature of the occupation in itself, are of a character which would justify the imputation that they are among the predisposing causes of the excessive mortality of the soldier by pulmonary disease[1].

I have already given their opinion as to the true causes of this contrast.

4. I have lately had occasion to examine into the distribution of phthisis in certain districts of Manchester and Salford, and have ascertained that in every case the parts of these districts most affected by the disease are the close courts and alleys, the shut-in streets, and especially the back-to-back houses.

[1] *Report of Commissioners on the Sanitary State of Army,* 1858.

5th and lastly. We may take an entirely different method of proof and we can show that wherever, in different parts of the world, there is an abundance of fresh air in the dwellings of the people, there is to be found a comparative immunity from the disease, even though most of the other surroundings are, in a sanitary point of view, almost as bad as they can be.

On the whole I think it may be regarded as fully proved that the breathing of air rendered foul by previous respiration is one of the conditions required to enable the bacillus of tubercle to take root and to grow in the lungs of human beings. Similar evidence is also forthcoming as to its influence upon animals—horses, cows, monkeys, etc.

It is important then to inquire what are the ingredients in respired air that are thus so potent for evil.

We can of course easily answer for one of them; and that one might be supposed sufficient to account for all the facts that have now been brought forward. I mean the tubercle bacillus itself. This must needs be present in such air, or the disease would not arise. It must come originally from the body of some tuberculous patient. It may have come directly from the breath, since it has been found in the watery vapour exhaled from the lungs of such persons; but it is more probably mixed up with the dust in the air, forming one of the innocent looking motes that dance in a sunbeam. It may have been at some time or other derived from the dried up excretions of some poor consumptive, by its inherent vitality outliving its victim; but the strange part of the story is that the micro-organism cannot do its work unless it is assisted by the presence of other impurities. We cannot doubt that the creature is given out into well-ventilated, as well as into badly aerated spaces, and yet so far as we know it never communicates the disease in the former case.

How is it that in the wards of a consumptive hospital, or in the sick rooms of well-ventilated houses, it never attacks the attendants? Even in the confined dwellings of the poor, direct contagion, in this country at any rate, is a very rare event; and where drainage and ventilation are good I have never heard of nor seen any case of direct transmission, even where there has been ample opportunity for breath to infect breath, as in the case of husband and wife or sisters sleeping together.

So far as we know the only other components of expired air that could have any effect in enhancing the virulence of the bacillus are the carbonic acid, the aqueous vapour, and the organic matter that it contains in excess. But all these substances must be present under the circumstances already spoken of, in which there is yet no direct transference of the disease. How, then, can these facts be reconciled with the overwhelming evidence that air rendered foul by respiration is one of the most powerful agents in producing consumption.

The explanation given by Dr Koch is (1) the need for some preliminary injury to the lungs in persons who are about to act the part of hosts to these parasitic organisms, some denudation of the mucous membrane of the lungs, or some injury to the elasticity of these organs ; and (2) the need for a plentiful supply of the infecting material.

The number of these microbes contained in the breath, even in advanced cases of phthisis is, as I can testify from repeated examinations, exceedingly small ; but, on the other hand, the dried sputum from such patients contains them in enormous quantities. " This sputum is not only ejected directly on to the floor, there to be dried up, to be pulverised, and to rise again in the form of dust, but a good deal of it dries on bed linen, articles of clothing, and especially pocket-handkerchiefs, which even the cleanliest of patients cannot help soiling with the dangerous infective material when wiping the mouth after expectoration ; and this also is subsequently scattered as dust."

I am doubtful myself how far this explanation would account for the exemption of the attendants of consumption hospitals from disease, and still more for the immunity conferred by residence upon well-drained porous soils.

It affords no reason for the diminution in the phthisis rate of Salisbury, for instance, by one half, after the introduction of proper drainage, and I am therefore inclined to believe that we have still not attained to a complete knowledge of the natural history of the microbe, and to venture the hypothesis that it may gain in virulence by a short sojourn outside the body, in the presence of organic compounds favourable to its existence, and contained either in impure ground air or else in air rendered foul by respiration. Experiments need to be made on this point.

In this case the bacillus of tubercle would fall into the same category as the microbe of enteric fever and cholera, and, whilst scarcely at all infective from person to person, it would gain the power of reproducing the disease by a sojourn for a shorter or longer time in some medium favourable to its development. If high temperatures are absolutely needed for its existence, I am inclined to think that it would find them in some nook or corner in the common kitchens and living-rooms inhabited by many of the poor inhabitants of our towns.

It is possible that all the components of expired air except the oxygen may take part in sustaining the existence of the microbe. I do not know whether the action upon it of carbonic acid has yet been ascertained, but it seems probable, from its continued existence in decomposing fluids, that it is one of those bacilli whose life is fostered by this vapour. We can see at once also that aqueous vapours charged with organic matter would be eminently fitted to sustain its existence. The nature of the organic matter contained in the breath is not yet fully ascertained ; it is probably partly gaseous and partly solid. I have myself examined it microscopically in a good many cases, both in health and disease, and have ascertained the quantity exhaled under various conditions. It certainly contains numerous solid particles ; some of it is simply disintegrated organised material, some dried up epithelial scales, and in some diseases, as in measles and whooping cough and phthisis, the specific organisms of the disease.

Its quantity is indeed very small; I found that only about 0·2 of a gramme is excreted per diem by healthy adults, or 0·4 gramme per metre of expired air; but this is 500 times as much as Dr de Chaumont found in the outer air, and when condensed upon solid bodies it often forms a perceptible foully smelling film ; and we know further from Dr Hammond's experiments that it is virulently poisonous, and it would probably sustain the life of the bacillus, though I am not aware of any direct experiments on this point[1].

[1] This surmise was afterwards confirmed. See Paper 6, Sect. III. p. 159.

We are now in a position to state the measures that are needed for the prevention of this terrible scourge of our population, and they may be thus briefly enumerated :

1. As far as possible the disinfection or destruction of the phthisical expectoration.

2. The discouragement of marriage between phthisical individuals.

3. The prevention of irritating dusts in workshops, or at any rate the adoption of means for sweeping them away from the mouths of workpeople, as is now almost universally done in the workshops of Sheffield.

4. The discouragement of stooping or confined postures during labour.

5. The better drainage of impervious soils, and the cleansing away of all kinds of filth.

6. The provision of thorough ventilation by night and day, not only in workshops, offices, warehouses, and factories, but also in the dwellings of both rich and poor, and in the streets and crowded alleys in which the latter live.

By the adoption of some such means as these I firmly believe that, in the course of time, we should see the present frightful mortality from consumption greatly diminished, and, although those measures could probably be only partially carried out, every effort in the right direction would be rewarded by some improvement in the death-rate, not only from consumption, but also from other diseases, and especially diseases of the lungs.

(3) CONSUMPTION, A " FILTH DISEASE[1] "

Reprinted from THE LANCET, *January* 1, 1898

SIR JOHN SIMON, in his admirable account of the class of complaints which he brands as " filth diseases," attributes them mainly
to two " gigantic evils " in the sanitary government of England :
" First, the omission (whether through neglect or through want
of skill) to make due removal of refuse matters, solid and liquid,
from inhabited places " ; and, " second, the licence which is
permitted to cases of dangerous infectious disease to scatter abroad
the seeds of their infection." He calls attention especially to the
class of " diarrhœal " diseases, such as diarrhœa and dysentery,
cholera, and enteric fever, and he regards the last-named as " the
very type and quintessence " of all the diseases which are attributable to filth. He says : " Though sometimes by covert
processes which I will afterwards explain, yet far oftener in the
most glaring way, it apparently has an invariable source in that
which of filth is the filthiest ; that apparently its infection runs
its course, as with successive inoculations from man to man, by
the instrumentality of the molecules of excrement which man's
filthiness lets mingle in his air and food and drink[2]." " There
are houses, there are groups of houses, there are whole villages,
there are considerable sections of towns, there are even entire and
not small towns, where general slovenliness in everything which
relates to the removal of refuse matter, slovenliness which in very
many cases amounts to utter bestiality of neglect, is the local
habit[3]."

Phthisis is not included in the list of " filth diseases " and the
omission was certainly intentional ; for whilst Sir John Simon
admits that foulness of air due to non-removal of the volatile
refuse of the human body is strictly within the physiologist's
definition of filth, yet, for the purpose of the report, the question
of overcrowding is set aside as distinct, and the word " filth " is

---

[1] A paper read at a meeting of the Bournemouth Medical Society on Nov. 10th ,
1897.
[2] *Public Health Reports*, vol. II. p. 459.   [3] *Ibid.* p. 463.

used only in that sense which suggests subject matter for sewers and scavenging. Notwithstanding this arbitrary definition, however, it may be contended that, in spite of all reservations, phthisis comes rightly within the class of filth diseases and the eminent writer of the report would probably be one of the first to acknowledge this. What, in fact, can be conceived as more fitted to come within the designation of filth, than the loathsome excretions from the lungs of phthisical patients? And what can better illustrate " utter bestiality of neglect " than the habit of voiding these excretions on the floors, or on the ground, of any place in which these patients may find themselves? The material of this expectoration contains, as is well known, myriads of the " seeds of infection." If this falls upon congenial soil it retains its vitality for long periods of time, even increasing in virulence if it is allowed to remain in this environment long enough for fresh colonies of the microbe to form. It may also dry up, may become powdered into tuberculous dust, and may then be wafted into the air, to be breathed into the lungs of susceptible persons, or to be deposited in milk, or in other foods, and may thus pass into the bodies of children, or of delicate persons predisposed to the reception of the disease. In one or another of these ways it comes strictly within the description given of a filth disease ; and in its effects it is infinitely more deadly than enteric fever, the " type and quintessence " of these disorders.

There are, in fact, many points of resemblance between tuberculous disease and enteric fever. The specific organism in each is a bacillus, remarkably long-lived in suitable surroundings, but easily deprived of its virulence by the action of sunlight. They are both " facultative saprophytes "—that is, though they are ordinarily parasites, they can exist, and even grow, outside the body in the presence sometimes of very small portions of organic matter. Neither disease is directly infectious. They both spread by means of the excretions from the body : phthisis chiefly by the intervention of " tuberculous dust," conveyed into the lungs by the medium of the air, enteric fever chiefly in drinking-water, by which means it passes into the intestines. Both diseases may, however, be conveyed either by air or by articles of food or drink.

It is not necessary to lay stress upon the similarity between

the lesions produced by these diseases, but it may be incidentally
pointed out that Villemin showed that tuberculosis shares with
syphilis, glanders, and enteric fever, the character of forming
" caseous " material. In his Gulstonian Lectures on Tubercle, also,
Dr Southey showed that typhoid lymphomata are very like tubercle
both in their composition, and their course, affecting similar parts
and leading to similar lesions. He places tubercle between cancer
and these other lymphomata. It is significant of the likeness
between phthisis and enteric fever, in respect of their derivation
from filth, that in this country both complaints have greatly declined in frequency, since the general improvement of drainage
and water-supply. In the last sixty years, phthisis has been
reduced to one-third of its former prevalence, and enteric fever to
one-fourth or less.

It is of so much importance that the connexion between phthisis
and filth should be clearly recognised, that it will be well to
advert briefly to the other evidence which is forthcoming to prove
the fact. This evidence is of two kinds—(*A*) statistical and
(*B*) experimental.

(*A*) *The statistical evidence.* 1. The returns of the Registrar-
General prove that phthisis has declined from over 3800 per
1,000,000 in 1838 to 1380 in 1894. This is a reduction of about
2500 per 1,000,000 annually or a saving of an army of 75,000 lives
in a year, or nearly three-quarters of a million in a decade. This
great improvement has probably been brought about mainly by
the better hygienic conditions of the people, especially as
regards sub-soil drainage, better dwellings, cleanliness, food
and clothing, etc.—in other words, by a diminution in the
amount of filth of various kinds. 2. This view is supported
by an analysis of these returns, showing the distribution of the
disease in overcrowded, unsanitary areas ; and by its incidence
upon certain portions of our large towns, its chosen sites being the
crowded, shut-in courts and alleys, the back-to-back houses, and
the one- or two-roomed tenements, where all kinds of filth, but
especially air-sewage, abound. 3. That this incidence of the
disease is not due simply to poverty, or to the poor constitutions
of the inhabitants, or to bad food, or exposure to the elements, or

to climate, is amply proved by the army and navy returns from
all parts of the world. These returns refer exclusively to men who
have been chosen from amongst the general population expressly
for their health and strength ; and it has been proved by Dr Welch
and others that they are less hereditarily predisposed to the
disease than the rest of the community. The report of the Army
Sanitary Commission shows that, in soldiers, the excessive mortality from phthisis was mainly due to the " bad ventilation and
the imperfect drainage of the barracks " in which they were
compelled to live, at all the stations to which these British troops
were sent. Similar conclusions are also to be drawn from the
Navy Medical Returns. 4. That the disease is not due, however,
to ordinary filth is sufficiently proved by the immunity of the
fishermen of St Kilda and of the St Lawrence River, who live in
vile surroundings, their huts being more like pig-sties than human
habitations ; and the same fact comes out in the history of many
a savage tribe. 5. A specific form of impurity is needed ; and
that this impurity is the peculiarly nasty product of phthisical
expectoration is clearly shown by the statistics relating to the
German nursing orders, collected and published by Dr Cornet.
No one studying these statistics can fail to come to the conclusion
that infection from the sick to the healthy had taken place, through
the medium of tuberculous dust, produced by the drying up and
grinding into powder of the excretions of tuberculous people.
The special incidence of the disease upon the novices, employed
to sweep the floors, would almost suffice by itself to point to its
source of origin. 6. But there are indications in these, and other
statistics, that the specific germ needs a special food and environment, either to preserve its existence, or to enhance its virulence.
The dirty, ill-lighted, ill-ventilated convent cells were evidently
peculiarly favourable to the tubercle bacillus ; and a similar conclusion must be formed from the report of the Army Sanitary
Commission, and from the many other returns from public institutions, prisons, reformatories, etc., which are given by Parkes in
his work on Hygiene, by Hirsch in his *Medical Geography* and
by others. 7. Lastly, statistics compiled by Bowditch and
Buchanan, by the Registrar General for Scotland, by Haviland
and others, show the influence upon the virulence of the disease

germ of emanations from a badly drained, impervious subsoil. These observations show at least the probability that certain special forms of impurity have an influence in promoting the infectiveness of the specific germ.

(*B*) *The experimental evidence.* Experimental researches have added weight to the conclusions to be drawn from statistics. (*a*) We have the observations of Villemin, Schottelius, and others to show that tuberculous material inhaled with the breath, or ingested in food, or in milk, will convey the disease to animals, and that it can also be inoculated under the skin. These researches show at any rate that this form of filth can produce the disease. (*b*) Professor Koch also, as the result of his exhaustive inquiries, came to the conclusion that tuberculous sputum dried up, and ground into dust, is the most common and most potent of all forms of infective material; and on a review of all the facts it is difficult to frame any other opinion. Cornet, indeed, by researches subsequent to those already mentioned, may be said to have proved this point by inoculating guinea-pigs with the dust from rooms, etc., and thus producing tuberculosis. (*c*) Experimental evidence is likewise forthcoming to indicate the nature of the special organic impurity which keeps alive the bacillus of tubercle. By means of some researches carried out in the years 1889 and 1890, with the assistance of Professor Dreschfeld, of Owens College, Manchester, I was able to show that the air of a poor cottage in Ancoats, with poor ventilation and undrained basement, in which several cases of phthisis had occurred, was able to preserve unchanged the virulence of tuberculous sputum for two or three months at least, but that the same sputum, exposed freely to air and light, in a hospital for phthisical patients, and also in a well-lighted, well-drained, and well-ventilated house, soon lost the power of communicating the disease to guinea-pigs by inoculation. A further research, carried on in 1894 in conjunction with Professor Delépine, proved that less than two days' exposure to air and light, with only one hour of sunshine, was sufficient to destroy the virulent power of tuberculous sputum, when it was exposed in a clean, well-drained, well-lighted house. Evidently, in the air of the Ancoats cottage, there must have been some form of organic

impurity favourable to the life of the bacillus. (*d*) During the
present year (1897) I have been able to demonstrate the character
of some of the substances thus capable of promoting the vitality
of these " seeds of infection." A vast number of substances have
been tried as cultivation media of the bacillus ; and Beck and
Proskauer have shown that, in the presence of glycerine, most
nitrogenous bodies are capable of sustaining its growth at the body
temperature. No attempt, however, seems to have been made
to test, in this respect, the influence of the substances most likely
to be met with by the organism, in its usual habitats, and at
ordinary temperatures. From a review of the statistical evidence,
it seemed most probable that some form of impurity, commonly
present in the air of unsanitary dwellings, would be likely to prove
a favourable medium of cultivation. A series of experiments was
therefore undertaken with the object of testing this point[1]. The
materials chosen for trial were : the condensed vapour from (1)
healthy breath ; (2) phthisical breath ; (3) cellar air (Southampton) ; (4) cellar air (Bournemouth) ; (5) a weaver's shed (Blackburn) ; and (6) pure ground air. These fluids were all carefully
sterilised and various substances were used as the supporting
medium upon which to sow the seed, such as simple glycerine agar,
potato, pure filter-paper, lining wall-paper. All these substances
were also sterilised and kept soaked in the fluids mentioned. All
the fluids proved to be excellent cultivating media, with or without
the addition of a small percentage of glycerine. (*e*) These experiments were carried on at temperatures of from 35° to 37° C. ; but
they were all repeated at a temperature of about 20° C., in order
to learn whether the usual conditions of many cottage homes
would suffice to keep the bacillus alive in these media. In a large
proportion of instances these latter experiments were also fairly
successful ; and it was thus proved that the virus of tubercle could
be kept alive, and could even grow, under these conditions. There
is now certainly nothing extraordinary in these results. Professor
Koch indeed asserted, on the basis of his own experiments, that
the bacillus of tubercle is a true parasite and that it could only be
cultivated at, or near, the temperature of the human body ; that

---

[1] This research was communicated to the Royal Society on Nov. 25th, 1897
(see *Proceedings of the Royal Society*; Paper 6, Sect. III. p. 159 in this volume).

it could not therefore have a saprophytic existence or live and grow at the ordinary temperatures of cottage dwellings. Other observers, however, notably Sir Hugh Beevor, Dr Kanthack, and Professor Delépine, have succeeded in cultivating the microbe on potato at comparatively low temperatures; and, as mentioned above, I have myself been successful with the media which I have employed. It may then be now regarded as certain that the bacillus can grow outside the body, whenever it can get hold of a sufficiently impure soil, and whenever its activity is not interfered with by the adverse conditions of abundant air and daylight. The filth-origin of the germ of phthisis and the sustaining influence of external filth upon its further growth may therefore be taken as proved.

The conclusion, that phthisis is a filth disease, is not likely to pass without protest from those cleanly people, whose families have suffered from the complaint. They will feel it to be a slur upon their reputation, and will ask wherefore it should come nigh their wholesome dwellings ? The truth is that both enteric fever and phthisis have the power of operating at a distance. Sir John Simon says with reference to the former : " Filth does not only infect where it stands, but can transmit its infective power afar by certain appropriate channels of conveyance. ... Thus it has again and again happened that an individual house, with every apparent cleanliness and luxury, has received the contagion of enteric fever through some unguarded drain inlet; or that numbers of such houses have simultaneously received the infection, as an epidemic, in places where the drain inlets in general have been subject to undue air-pressure from within the sewer. It has again and again happened, that households, while themselves without sanitary reproach, have received the contagium of enteric fever through some nastiness affecting (perhaps at a considerable distance) the common water-supply of the district in which they are[1]." He instances the case of Windsor, when the highest persons in the land were affected ; and the cases of Croydon, and Worthing. Much the same may be said of phthisis, from which complaint many have suffered whose houses are above reproach, though it may be doubted whether there are not many, even of the

[1] *Collection of Works* (Memorial Volume), p. 465.

luxurious homes of the rich, where air-sewage is not merely allowed
to remain, but where it is even closely stored up by the precautions taken against cold and draught. Even where there is an
abundance of fresh air and sunlight, is it certain that the inmates
of these perfectly hygienic houses never visit places where the
specific forms of filth are to be found in abundance, and in full
possession of all their virulence? What are we to say of many
of the places frequented by these otherwise happily situated
individuals? What of the constantly attended places of public
resort? What of the theatres, concert halls, assembly rooms,
churches, chapels, etc.?

Theatres, as at present constructed, are often mere death-
traps to delicate, susceptible people. These so-called temples of
the Thespian art are often charged with many different forms of
pathogenic microbes, ready to flourish into disease when they
meet with congenial soil. They are nightly filled with people, some
of whom at least are in one or another of the stages of phthisis, and
though perhaps many of them are too well bred to expectorate
upon the floors, others are not so particular, and nearly all carry
about with them handkerchiefs laden with tuberculous material.
The halls and passages and galleries of these places, and even their
auditoria, are seldom if ever visited by the rays of sunlight; and
their atmospheres are overcharged with carbonic acid and am-
moniacal or sulphurous vapours. They are imperfectly ventilated,
chiefly in many cases by the spent and disease-laden air from the
stage and wings, where the employés are still more liable to be in
advanced stages of phthisis; and where they are still less likely
to abstain from spitting upon the floors, scenery, etc. They are
true hotbeds and forcing grounds in which may be kept alive, and
even cultivated, the germs of tuberculous and other diseases.

Concert halls and assembly rooms are in little better case than
theatres, in respect of their appliances for ventilation, for cleanliness, and for the admission of sunlight.

What again shall we say of churches and chapels and other
places of public worship? Is it not notorious how badly they
are ventilated and how little their " dim religious light " can do
to disinfect the germs of disease? Let anyone, gifted with an
ordinary sense of smell, or who knows what fresh air means, enter

almost any of these places for public worship, even after only a short service, and let him describe the atmosphere he will meet with on entering. It is charged with " air-sewage " of the vilest quality, the imperfectly removed emanations from hundreds or thousands of human bodies. There is probably less visible filth than in places of amusement ; but, even here, there can be no doubt that there is plenty of tuberculous dust floating about in the air ; and the conditions it finds there are well calculated to keep it alive, and to preserve its virulence. Here again, therefore, we have an important source of danger to the individuals whose case we are now considering. There is also danger in closely shut up, and badly ventilated, vehicles such as omnibuses and railway carriages ; and, in fine, we have not far to look for sources of phthisis in most of the haunts of ordinary so-called civilised life. It cannot be said, therefore, that any direct blame attaches to the families of those who have fallen victims to phthisis. The opprobrium rests rather with the supreme health authorities, and with the general public, for allowing places of public resort to remain in such a condition as to be a serious source of danger to their frequenters. It is a public scandal that places of amusement, and our temples of worship, should be allowed to remain without adequate ventilation and without frequent and periodical purification.

It is possible that, owing to the terms in which I have described the dangers arising from places of public assembly, I may be accused of attempting to increase the " scare " of infection which at present undoubtedly possesses the public mind, but this is very far from my intention. I believe that in temperate climates direct infection from patients is one of the rarest events. It is only when tuberculous filth is scattered about in places fitted to keep alive the bacillus, that infection becomes probable ; and it is therefore against the retention of gross impurities in the air that the above remarks have been written. I have elsewhere given my reasons for concluding that in well-kept, cleanly, well-aerated, and well-lighted, dwellings[1] there is little, if any, danger of infection from phthisical persons. On the other hand, I believe strongly in the danger of infected, insanitary houses, and even infected areas, and it has been owing to that conviction that I have ventured

[1] *On the Limits of Infection by Tubercle* (Cornish, Manchester).

to raise a protest against the filthy habits of communities, and against the vile conditions of our public assembly rooms, under which infection from phthisis is only too likely to take place.

It will be gathered from what has been said that, in my opinion, it is not the person of the phthisical subject that is to be dreaded, but the conditions under which he lives. It is true that, like the typhoid fever patient, he is the source and origin of the infective material, but he is not himself directly infectious. In the case of enteric fever, it is well known that if proper care is taken to disinfect, and to dispose of, the excreta, there is no risk of infection to the attendants ; and the same immunity can be claimed under this condition for the nurses of phthisical persons.

The measures to be adopted, in order to prevent the spread of phthisis, are indeed very similar to those required for staving off an epidemic of enteric fever ; with this difference, that instead of paying especial attention to drains and sewers, and to the condition of the drinking-water, it is the purification of the air, the admission of sunlight, the drainage of the sub-soil, the provision of damp-proof courses and concrete basements, that must be chiefly attended to for the prevention of phthisis. The means which are used, and which have been to a great extent successful, for the suppression of enteric fever are—(a) notification of disease, (b) disinfection of excreta, (c) hospital treatment, and (d) general sanitary measures. Similar methods, with certain modifications to suit the differences between the conditions of the disorders, must be adopted for the suppression of phthisis. Thus (a) the notification of phthisis can hardly be made compulsory, as in the case of enteric fever. Phthisis usually runs a much more chronic course than typhoid fever ; it is not unfrequently difficult to make an accurate diagnosis ; and the announcement of its presence would be regarded by many as a blot upon the family escutcheon, especially among the upper classes of society. Notification amongst these classes would indeed be almost useless ; since no medical officer would interfere with the private medical practitioner, and we may be sure that for their own sakes these families would take every care to prevent the spread of infection. In Manchester, a plan of procedure was formulated a few years ago, at a meeting, called together at my suggestion, of the medical officers of the

Hospital for Consumption, some of the physicians of the Royal Infirmary, and Dr Tatham, then the medical officer of health of Manchester. It was proposed that the medical officer of health should send to the medical men then present, and to any others willing to carry out the modified notification, post-cards addressed to himself, which should be filled up with the names and addresses of phthisical patients, in whom the disease had advanced as far as excavation, or in whose sputum bacilli had been detected. Only those cases were to be reported which were likely to spread infection owing to the state of their dwellings, or to want of means, or of will, to disinfect. These cards were to be countersigned by the patients themselves. On his part, the medical officer of health promised to send to these people carefully drawn up papers of instructions, stating the precautions to be taken with the sputum, or other excreta, and directions as to ventilation and admission of sunlight. He also offered to disinfect free of charge any dwelling likely to be a source of danger. This plan of campaign was adopted, both in Manchester and in Salford; and was to some extent carried out not only in these towns but in the surrounding district. It was also unanimously approved of by the north-western branch of the Association of Medical Officers of Health[1]. (*b*) Destruction of the bacillus in the excreta must be carried out by 1 per 500 solutions of corrosive sublimate, by fire, or by sluicing away the already disinfected excreta into the sewers. Infected houses must be treated by brushing over all surfaces with 1 per cent. solutions of chloride of lime, according to Professor Delépine's directions. (*c*) Although, in so chronic an ailment, hospital accommodation cannot be provided for all the cases likely to require isolation, yet it would undoubtedly be a great benefit both to the sufferers themselves, and to the general community, if all who were without proper lodging and accommodation, or who were unable themselves to take proper precautions, could be received for treatment into fitting homes. May we not hope that, in the near future, local authorities will see the importance of establishing, in connexion with fever hospitals, wards for the reception of all such cases? It is much to be regretted that the

---

[1] A somewhat similar scheme has also for the last year or two been carried out in New York. (See *Report of the Medical Officer of Health.*)

funds, formerly so lavishly provided for the segregation of lepers, are not now available for the treatment of the strictly analogous disease, tuberculosis. (*d*) The last of the measures to be directed against the spread of these " filth diseases "—namely, sanitary reform—is also probably the most important. We know how efficient it has been against enteric fever, and it is probable that when it is once fairly directed against tuberculosis it will be equally successful. Already the simple measures of improved drainage, better house accommodation, better food, etc., which have diminished the death-rate from enteric fever, have had some effect upon the mortality from phthisis, reducing it by nearly two-thirds, as I have already pointed out. Some more special means will, however, have to be adopted if the remaining third of this mortality is to be abolished. Particular attention will have to be paid, as we have seen, to the condition of the air in all places of public assembly; and a much higher standard of ventilation will have to be ensured in all workshops, weaving sheds, and in all rooms occupied by working people. It is much to be desired that the standard, recently proposed by the Home Office Committee on Cotton Cloth Factories, of which I was a member, could be applied to all places where manual labour is carried on. Again, " air-sewage " must be promptly carried away, or destroyed, in all the densely populated recesses of our towns ; and, in order that the natural enemies of the tubercle-bacillus—fresh air and sunlight—may have free scope to act, local authorities will everywhere be obliged to carry out extensive works of reconstruction, and will have to put in force the strongest powers they now possess, for preventing the pollution of the atmosphere by smoke or noxious vapours ; they must open out all confined areas, must destroy all insanitary house property, and must provide ample lung-space in the shape of public parks and playgrounds. It would be well also, if all towns would follow the enlightened policy of Liverpool and London, and obtain powers for securing that an adequate space shall be left around all houses or buildings in the future ; and that ground air shall be excluded from buildings, by efficient concrete basements, damp-proof courses, etc. Owing to the recognition of the fact that enteric fever can be stamped out by attention to the water-supply, and by the proper disposal of abdominal excreta, this disease has now come to be regarded as entirely preventable ; and its presence is felt to be an opprobrium upon the sanitary management of the community. If it could be made plain to men's minds that phthisis is likewise essentially a " filth disease," and if the means of disposing of the " air sewage," from which it springs, could be clearly shown to the people, its presence as an endemic in any community would quickly come to be regarded as an opprobrium, and the disease would soon be as great a rarity as leprosy.

(4) A CRUSADE AGAINST TUBERCULOSIS

Reprinted from THE MEDICAL CHRONICLE, *September*, 1898

A NATIONAL movement for the limitation, and ultimately the abolition, of tuberculosis has recently been commenced; and, judging from the support that it has received from the Royal Colleges of Physicians and Surgeons, from the most eminent members of the medical profession, and from others who rank as the highest in the land, we may fairly hope for a successful result.

It may, perhaps, be interesting to trace the events which have led to this movement, and to point out the direction that it may be expected to take.

The first intimation of the preventability of phthisis probably came from the results published by the Commission on the Sanitary State of the Army, in the year 1858; results which were ably commented on by the late Sir William Farr, and which both pointed out some of the common causes of the disease, and also indicated the means of prevention by thorough drainage of the soil and free ventilation.

The evidence collected by Dr Edward Parkes, and published in his great work on hygiene, added force to the conclusions of this Commission, and spurred on to action those who were responsible for the public health.

The discoveries of Dr Bowditch, in America, and of Dr Buchanan, in England, also showed the possibility of controlling the spread of phthisis by means of sub-soil drainage.

The probability of infection by tubercular products, when inhaled, was clearly shown by Villemin, Schottelius, and others; and the conditions under which such infection can take place were shadowed forth by the Report of the Collective Investigation Committee of the British Medical Association, by my own researches on Tubercular Infective Areas (Epidemiological Society)[1], by those of Dr Niven, and of Dr Flick of Philadelphia.

[1] See Sect. IV. (1), p. 176.

The strongest impetus to the full recognition of the preventability of tuberculosis was, however, given by Dr Koch's discovery of the microbic nature of the disease ; and so strong an impression was made upon the public mind, especially on the Continent, as to the contagion of phthisis, that there was, and still is, danger that the conditions of such infection, and the true sources of safety, might be overlooked, and that phthisical persons might, without reason, come to be regarded with as much dread as lepers.

Strength was given to the scare of infection by Dr Cornet's statistics respecting the Nursing Orders in Germany, and by his researches showing the virulence of the dust upon the walls of rooms that had been occupied by phthisical persons.

Viewed impartially, however, these very researches might have inspired confidence in the disinfecting power of light and air as a protection against infection ; for they clearly proved the immunity of hospital wards where these conditions were present.

Other observations, amongst which I may perhaps be allowed to refer to those conducted by myself, along with Professors Dreschfeld and Delépine[1], also indicated the virulence of tubercular sputum, under certain conditions of soil, light, and air, and its complete disinfection by air in the presence of sunlight.

The attention of most of the medical practitioners throughout the world was, however, almost wholly taken up by attempts to cause all consumptives to disinfect and dispose of their sputum before it could change into tuberculous dust, and thus pollute the air with infectious material.

It is not surprising that this course should have commended tself, in the first place, to those who are interested in the public health. It is obvious that if we could secure, by chemical means, the destruction of the virus on its ejection from the body, infection from this, the most common of all sources of infection, might be expected to die out.

It was speedily perceived, however, that the numerous cases of concealed or unsuspected phthisis, or the presence of ignorant or careless individuals affected by the disease, would completely frustrate the attempts to destroy the deadly seed by ordinary disinfectants ; hence there speedily arose a cry for the notification

[1] *Proceedings of the Royal Society*, vol. LVI.

of cases of phthisis, and for the segregation of certain of them in
sanatoria or hospitals for consumption. Few persons were disposed
to trust to the natural disinfection by fresh air and sunlight;
although these agents would act automatically and without
official intervention.

I believe that Manchester has the honour of being the first town
in the kingdom both to suggest, and partially to carry out, measures
for the prevention of phthisis.

Seven years ago an informal meeting was held, in my house,
of certain members of the staffs of the Manchester Royal Infirmary
and of the Hospital for Consumption; and Dr Tatham, then
Medical Officer of Health for Manchester, was also present.
A resolution was carried that it was desirable that the houses of
consumptive patients at these institutions should be periodically
disinfected; and, mainly owing to the courage and public spirit
of Dr Tatham, it was determined that in any cases notified to
him by members of these staffs, the occupants should have the
houses thoroughly purified free of cost.

This undertaking was carried out for some time; but was then
discontinued, in order that experiments as to the most efficient
methods of disinfection might be made by Professor Delépine of
the Owens College. These researches revealed that the best
disinfectant against the bacillus of tubercle is a one per cent.
solution of chloride of lime. But I am not aware that the undertaking was resumed after this result was made known.

This effort was not the only one made in this direction. Papers,
covering the whole method of procedure, were published on the
subject; one by the Manchester and Salford Sanitary Association
entitled *A Campaign against Phthisis*, and others by Dr Niven
and myself, read before the Society of Medical Officers of Health
(North-Western Branch); and it was unanimously determined
by this body to carry out the views of the writers of these papers.

Shortly after this date, papers were read at the International
Medical Congress in London, by Dr Squire and myself, dealing
with the subject; and I am glad to remember that special stress
was laid upon " the need for general sanitary measures " in order to
produce " any large reduction in the mortality from tubercle."

Several papers dealing with the subject have since then

appeared in the medical journals from time to time[1]; but unquestionably to Mr Malcolm Morris belongs the honour of having stirred up the medical profession in London (by his "Tuberculosis Number" of the *Practitioner*), and, under Sir W. Broadbent's leadership, of having brought about the formation of a National League for the Suppression of Tubercle.

At the inaugural meeting, at Sir W. Broadbent's, Mr Malcolm Morris pointed out that other nations had been before Great Britain in starting similar measures of prevention of tuberculosis—notably France, Belgium, and the United States. Quite recently, also, Norway has proposed to legislate on the subject[2].

In the number of the *Practitioner* already mentioned, Dr Herman Biggs gives a full account of the means adopted in the city of New York for the prevention and restriction of pulmonary tuberculosis. The undertaking was commenced in a tentative manner as far back as the year 1893 ; and in 1897 legal force was given to these measures. They have already proved of great service, and will have to be carefully studied by the leaders of the movement now about to be carried out in England.

This brief review of the chief events which led to the present undertaking may, perhaps, suffice to show its importance and the widespread feeling of its necessity. It will now be desirable to indicate the directions in which effort will have to be made, in order to cope effectively with this formidable malady.

(1) It is important to ascertain the full extent of the evil that has to be dealt with ; and, to this end, a complete census of all persons suffering from the malady should be made.

(*a*) Notification of all classes of tubercular disease, as complete as possible, should be obtained ; but, as in New York, there should be no intervention between physician and patient in any tubercular case in which the intelligent practitioner may be trusted to give the simple instructions necessary to prevent the transmission of the disease to others. All the arrangements in New York for recording both cases and deaths, and the action taken in order

[1] "On Re-infection in Phthisie" (*Med. Chron.* October, 1892); "Leprosy and Tuberculosis" (*Lancet,* July 11, 1896); "The Consumption Scare" (*Med. Chron.* December, 1897, and *Lancet*).
[2] *Public Health,* vol. x. p. 430.

to prevent infection, will probably have to be closely followed in our own campaign against the disease.

(*b*) Similar returns as to the proportion of cattle affected by tubercular disease should be obtained. All herds of cattle will have to be thoroughly inspected, and tested by tuberculin, in order that we may know the exact degree of danger from this possible source of infection.

(2) Measures for the prevention of infection will have to be undertaken.

(*a*) Instructions as to the best means of destroying the sputum, and other discharges from tuberculous patients, will have to be widely circulated. Here again we shall have valuable assistance in the admirable leaflet on the subject, issued by the New York authorities. It is given at length by Mr Malcolm Morris, in his article in the *Fortnightly* for August, 1898.

(*b*) All the cases of tuberculosis reported to the authorities by their medical attendants as being in need of such help, will have to be visited in their homes by medical inspectors detailed for the purpose. They will give verbal directions and will decide upon the best course to be taken in each case.

(*c*) If the case is one which, in the judgment of the inspector, requires special hospital treatment, the fact must be reported to the authority, and the patient will have to be visited, as in New York, by a special inspector, who will determine, by physical and bacteriological examination, whether the case is tubercular. He will also have to decide whether the patient is in circumstances which prevent him from receiving proper care and medical attendance, and whether he is a source of danger to others. Under such circumstances he will endeavour to have him removed to some special hospital, and will take measures to have his house properly disinfected.

(*d*) The provision of suitable hospitals will have to be another very important aim of the League. At the present time, with the exception of a few hospitals for consumption in London, and still fewer in other parts of the kingdom, the workhouse hospitals are the only refuges to which these poor patients can be sent.

At the inaugural meeting of the Society it was mentioned that one of its objects would be the establishment of suitable " open-air sanatoria " in different parts of the kingdom.

It would be well for the attainment of this object if we could follow the example of Norway, where Dr Nansen has just succeeded in getting possession of about £100,000, which had previously been set aside for the use of lepers. We have even less danger than the Norwegians from leprosy ; and there must be enormous sums somewhere in the country, formerly devoted to " leper-houses," but which are now diverted to other uses, and which might most legitimately be transferred to the treatment of the strictly kindred disorder, tuberculosis.

(e) The disinfection of infected houses, whether before or after the death of the occupier, should be, as it is in Manchester, carried out at the expense of the municipality. In New York the process is called " renovation," not disinfection. Dr Biggs remarks—" This involves the application of simple, and, in tene-ment houses, inexpensive measures, *i.e.* scrubbing painted wood-work and floors with hot soda solution, and repainting, repapering, or rekalsomining the walls. ..."

" Where the consent of the owners can be obtained (and there is now but little difficulty in this) infected bedding, clothing, carpets, etc., are removed...to the disinfecting station, and disinfected by steam or destroyed, at the option of the owner, without expense to him."

(f) The danger of infection from tuberculous meat or milk must be averted by thorough supervision of all herds of cattle, by the control of the sale of tuberculous meat, by the gradual forma-tion of herds of non-tuberculous cattle, by the stringent regula-tion of dairies and milkshops, and by the boiling or Pasteurisation of all suspected milk.

Hitherto, as I have already pointed out, this seems to be all that has been attempted by the organisations in other countries ; but, if the disease is to be effectually restrained, much more than this will have to be carried out.

In spite of the best devised schemes of notification, many cases of tubercular disease will slip through the net ; there will remain many centres of infection in the unsanitary tenements which exist in all large towns ; and places of public assembly, such as theatres, churches, chapels, workshops, public-houses, etc., will still continue to be potent means of spreading the disease.

In addition to the other measures which have been enumerated, the British Society for the Suppression of Tuberculosis will have to promote all those measures of general sanitary reform which have already diminished the disease by nearly two-thirds in this country, and which may be expected to effect still further improvement in this direction.

I trust, also, that they will suggest special measures for the cleansing and disinfection of all places of public assembly ; for the ventilation and periodical cleansing of workshops ; for the prevention of overcrowding in schools ; and for their better ventilation and purification.

Briefly stated, the aims of a Society for the Prevention of Tuberculosis must be :

(1) The accumulation of information as to the amount and localisation of the disease.

(2) The dissemination of information amongst the general public, and especially amongst the poorer classes, with regard to the precautions to be taken to prevent its spread.

(3) The enlightenment of local authorities as to their duties in regard to its prevention, especially respecting the milk and the meat supply, the disinfection of dwellings, and the examination of tuberculous products, free of cost to individuals.

(4) The promotion of improved building byelaws in all the chief towns in the country, and the encouragement of the inhabitants to obtain more civic "lung-space" in the shape of parks and open pleasure-grounds.

(5) The establishment of " open-air " sanatoria for the poor in certain well-chosen localities.

In order to carry out these objects it will probably be necessary to ask for the co-operation of all the branches of the British Medical Association ; to assist in the formation of branches of the Society in all the great centres of the population ; to endeavour to enlist in the service large bodies of workpeople and trades-unionists ; and to appoint lecturers who would deliver simple " health-lectures " on subjects likely to improve the general health of the population.

(5) THE NEED OF A STANDARD OF EFFICIENT VENTILATION IN ALL WORK-PLACES AND PLACES OF PUBLIC ASSEMBLY

Read before the State Section of the British Conference on Tuberculosis, 1901

IT is now universally acknowledged that the breathing of atmospheres laden with organic impurity, especially when this comes from respiratory sources, is closely associated with the spread of tubercular diseases of the lungs.

The evidence in support of this proposition is overwhelming. The prevalence of phthisis on badly drained or impervious soils, in densely populated neighbourhoods, in ill-ventilated workshops, dwellings, barracks, prisons, etc. ; its origin in certain tubercle-infected houses or areas ; in dusty, crowded, inefficiently ventilated places of public assembly ; all these circumstances tend to increase the death-rate from consumption, and they are all more or less connected with the one factor, the presence of air polluted with organic matter.

It is probable that the incidence of consumption upon communities living under one or another of the above-mentioned conditions is due to more than one influence.

(1) First and chief, we have in such places a greater probability that tubercle bacilli are present in the floating dust of the air.

(2) In such places also the bacillus retains its virulence for much longer periods of time than in comparatively pure air.

(3) In foul air these organisms are usually accompanied by numerous other pathogenic germs, whose office it is to make the entrance of the specific microbe more ready and easy.

(4) Add to these favouring facts the probability that the inhabitants of such localities are, for the most part, the very poorest, the worst nourished, and the least careful, members of the population ; and

(5) The extreme likelihood (though this is not yet proved)

that persons exposed for long periods of time to these adverse
conditions are less able to resist the attack of the enemy, when it
succeeds in obtaining an entrance.

Whatever may be the explanation of the facts, it is obvious
that one of the first duties of those who are organising the " campaign against phthisis " must be to get rid of these conditions so
favourable to the disease, in other words, to sweep away the " air
sewage " wheresoever this may be found.

Hitherto local sanitary authorities have turned their attention
chiefly to the disposal of water sewage ; but, when the account is
fairly made out, it will be found that impurities in the air have
exacted from communities a far heavier death toll than have
imperfections of drainage and water-supply. Compare, for
instance, the steady, relentless slaughter of more than half a million
persons every decade with the occasional epidemic death-rates
from cholera or enteric fever. The worst mortality from these
two diseases, in any one decade, never equalled this terrible
mortality ; a mortality which is constantly going on.

The only means of keeping the air of crowded places free from
a dangerous degree of impurity is that of sweeping it away constantly by currents of pure air, in other words, by copious " ventilation."

For dwelling rooms the standard of efficient ventilation has
been fixed by the masters of public health at 3000 cubic feet per
head per hour.

This standard depended originally upon an observation of the
late Dr R. Angus Smith, to the effect that the smell of organic
impurity in the air begins to be perceptible when the CO_2 of respiratory origin reaches 4 parts per 10,000, that is, if the outer air contains also 4 parts, when the total amount of CO_2 reaches 8 parts
per 10,000. He also noticed that when this limit was reached
such air often caused headache and general malaise.

Practical observations have confirmed this general statement ;
notably those of Wilson, who showed that, in certain cells of the
Portsmouth Convict Prison, of 614 cubic feet always occupied,
the CO_2 equalled 0·720 per 1000, and the prisoners remained
healthy and of good colour. In cells of 210 cubic feet, occupied
only at night by prisoners employed outside during the day, he

found 1·044 per 1000 of CO_2; the occupants were all pale and anæmic.

For safety's sake the permissible amount of respiratory CO_2 has been fixed at half the amount ascertained to be noxious, namely, at 2 parts per 10,000, and, seeing that about 0·6 of a cubic foot of CO_2 is exhaled, on the average, by human beings per head per hour, it is obvious that, to dilute this down to 0·2 parts per 1000 cubic feet, 3000 cubic feet per head must be admitted to a living room every hour.

It will be noted that in this calculation it has been taken for granted that the proportion of CO_2 is also a measure of the organic impurity in the air; but a little consideration will soon show that this cannot be always the case, for CO_2, as a gas, is rapidly diffusible; whilst the organic matter is particulate, and can thus only be swept away by sufficiently strong currents of wind.

Notwithstanding this fact the proportion of CO_2 may be taken as a very fair criterion of the efficiency of ventilation. Although, in stagnant air, the CO_2 may diffuse away and the organic impurity be left, by ventilation both of them are swept away together, and thus the CO_2 becomes a very fair standard for purposes of comparison between a good and bad system of ventilation.

In their inquiry into the ventilation of schools, Carnelly, Haldane and Anderson found a general relationship between the CO_2 and the organic impurity, so that a high carbon dioxide content is, as a rule, accompanied by a high organic matter content, and *vice versa.*

In a Home Office inquiry into the circumstances of humidified cotton weaving sheds, in which I took part, along with Sir H. Roscoe and the late Sir W. Roberts, we found that the amount of ventilation required by statute in these places was insufficient, and we recommended that, " as a measure of the respiratory impurity, no greater proportion than nine-tenths of a volume of CO_2 per 1000 volumes of air should be contained in the air of the sheds, and that the ventilating arrangements should be sufficient to secure the general attainment of this standard."

They said, " in fixing this standard, your Committee are aware that from a medical point of view this proportion may be considered too high. They have, however, suggested this limit, believing

that, if effectually carried out, a very great improvement in the
air of the sheds will be brought about, without laying any serious
burden on the trade, and, in fact, without asking for more to be
done than is now actually carried out voluntarily in well regulated
sheds. This limit will secure an amount of ventilation corresponding to about 2000 cubic feet per head per hour, and your
Committee believe that such a requirement would bring about a
material improvement in the health and comfort of the workers."

The proposal was accepted without opposition by both masters
and workpeople ; and in the ensuing session of Parliament it was
embodied, together with other suggestions, in the Cotton Cloth
Factories Act of 1897.

Sufficient time has not yet elapsed, since the passing of this
Act, to enable us to judge of its results ; but already, in his Report
to the Chief Inspector, in 1899, Mr Williams, the Inspector under
the Cotton Cloth Factories Acts, remarked that the scientific test
" has already led to a great improvement in the working conditions
of many thousands of operatives, and it has also done much to
promote an intelligent interest and a more exact knowledge on
the subject of ventilation."

He also gives a statement showing the results of tests made of
samples of air taken from the middle of sheds before and after the
improved means of ventilation were installed. These results are
shown in the table overleaf[1].

From this table it will be seen that, owing to the improvement
in the systems of ventilation introduced by the manufacturers,
the amount of respiratory impurity has, in most cases, been diminished by one half, and in some it is only one quarter of what it
was before the passing of the Act.

In a private letter, Mr Williams tells me that he has ascertained
from several managers of these reformed sheds that the health of
the operatives has been greatly improved, and that the sickness
rate is much smaller than before the improvements.

---

[1] In his Report for 1900, Mr Williams gives a more extended table, and also
figures, relating to the CO_2 in cotton-spinning mills, which show that where there
are no mechanical means of ventilation, the quantity of carbonic acid per 10,000
of air usually exceeds twenty volumes, an appalling amount, which must lead to
ill-health.

Table showing Results of Analyses of Samples of Air taken respectively before and after Improvement of Ventilating Arrangements in certain Cotton-Weaving Sheds.

Number of Comparison	Number of Volumes of CO₂ per 10,000 Volumes of Air.		Approximate Number of Volumes of CO₂ per 10,000, due to Respiration	
	Before Improvement	After	Before Improvement	After
(1)	12·0	7·1	8·0	3·1
(2)	10·8	8·2	6·8	4·2
(3)	14·7	7·1	10·7	3·1
(4)	15·3	6·6	11·3	2·6
(5)	10·9	7·0	6·9	3·0
(6)	13·0	8·2	9·0	4·2
(7)	13·2	7·8	9·2	3·8
(8)	15·4	7·6	11·4	3·6
(9)	11·7	6·4	7·7	2·4
(10)	14·4	7·7	10·4	3·7
(11)	11·3	6·4	7·3	2·4

The approximate number of Volumes of CO_2 per 10,000 ascribed to Respiration, given in the two last columns, are obtained by simply subtracting 4 (the usual normal amount of CO_2) from the two preceding columns.

When we consider the full meaning of these facts, it becomes the duty of all who are concerned with the health of our British workpeople, who are the " backbone " of the country, to see that the great benefits of the ventilation of all " work-places " should be secured to them as soon as possible.

The beneficial influence of the Cotton Factories Act of 1897 is at present only extended to the workers in " humidified cotton weaving factories "—to not more than about one hundred thousand male and female operatives ; but there are some millions of others who are now left to perform their arduous labour under the old conditions of insufficient air-supply.

There can be no doubt that if the same standard of ventilation were applied to all work-places, the health of the people who work in them would be benefited to at least the same extent, and that the prevalence of consumption amongst them would be reduced greatly.

Not only would these workers breathe purer air during their labour, and thus avoid the danger of infection during their work, but they would be taught the invigorating power of fresh air, and would find themselves unable to tolerate the close and polluted atmospheres of their own homes. They would learn to keep open their windows at night as well as in the day, and would thus escape the bugbear of " catching cold," which is now such a fertile source of many forms of ill-health.

Lastly, I would put in a plea for some regulation of the ventilation of all places of public assembly—theatres, concert rooms, churches, chapels, and rooms in which public meetings are held. There can be little doubt that consumption is kept up to its present high mark by the tuberculous dust which now circulates in the air-sewage of these places ; and it is high time that steps were taken to rid ourselves of this opprobrium.

I am aware that the chief objections that will be made to these propositions will be on the score of the expense of carrying them out.

Not only will some people deprecate putting manufacturers to the additional charges involved, but, if the methods employed are made the subject of Government inspection, the cost of payment of qualified inspectors will be a serious item in the balance sheet of the nation.

I would not make light of either of these difficulties ; but as regards the first, I would point out that, when the employers of labour realise the gain accruing through the better health of their workpeople, and when the operatives find out the improvement in health and efficiency due to better ventilation, both parties will voluntarily accept the improved conditions of labour ; and we may fairly hope that the trades unions will help on the beneficent work.

In this case there will be little need of additional inspectors, and thus one of the most important objections will fall to the ground.

The more difficult problem of securing better ventilation in places of public assembly, and, still more important, in shops and in the offices where many clerks are employed, must be left to the outside pressure of public opinion ; but when the great danger of infection, existing in these places, is made fully manifest to the minds of those who are involved in its meshes, there will arise a cry for protection against the risk which the keepers of these centres of infection will no longer be able to resist, and there will be a general demand for their better ventilation.

I venture, therefore, to propose the following resolution :

> " That the Council of the National Association for the Prevention of Tuberculosis be requested to impress upon all employers of labour, and upon the managers of all places of public assembly, the danger of polluted atmospheres, and the urgent need of efficient ventilation[1]."

[1] Carried *nem. con.* This resolution was brought up for consideration at a meeting of the Council and was forwarded to several Employers' Associations.

(6) DUTIES OF THE STATE IN REGARD TO TUBERCULOSIS

Address to the Manchester Medico-Ethical Association, October, 1912

I DO not think that the State should undertake the treatment of disease. It should rather turn attention in the direction of prevention. Indeed, the results of many other enterprises undertaken by the State or by municipal authorities prove that it is improbable in the highest degree that State officials can succeed in the treatment of tuberculosis as well as do at present the several voluntary agencies.

It is possible that the State may rightly concern itself with the medical treatment of its own employees, as in the Post Office or in the navy and army ; but, even for them, this work will probably be better carried out by men who are not under State supervision. Again, it will be said that the State necessarily provides medical treatment for those unfortunate persons who, owing to poverty, are, as paupers, entirely dependent upon the State ; and this is true. But who will say that the Poor Law medical service is a model of what medical treatment by the State ought to be ? Is not this very service an object lesson as to the results that are likely to follow when the State goes out of its province and tries to undertake the treatment of disease ? Notwithstanding the noble and self-sacrificing conduct of many Poor Law medical officers, this department of medical practice is undoubtedly the lowest and the worst. It is degrading to the doctor, and it is unwelcome to his patients. It is degrading to the doctor because he is compelled to attend people who have no confidence in him ; and it is unwelcome to the poor because the doctor is imposed upon them by the State, and because they have no choice as to whom they should have to attend them. If there be any one who doubts these statements let him read the report of the Poor Law Commission of 1909. He will find that it is full of evidence of the unsatisfactory nature of this sample of State interference with medical treatment.

I venture to affirm as deductions from this evidence,

(1) "That the present plan of medically assisting the poor under the Poor Law is not an efficient system[1].

(2) That in too many Unions outdoor medical relief begins and ends with a bottle of medicine, and that the bottle of physic is a very curse. It is responsible for what may be called the mortality of delay[2].

(3) That under the Poor Law there is practically no sanitary supervision of phthisis in the home of the patient. ....Phthisis cases are maintained in crowded, unventilated houses. It is not regarded as any part of the duty of the district medical officer to take any steps to prevent disease, either in the way of recurrence in the same patient, or in its spread to other persons[3].

From first to last, in short, the outdoor medical officers of the Poor Law have no conception of the public health point of view."

Much the same conclusions are reached when we consider the indoor treatment of paupers by the State; but on this point I will only quote a few passages from *The State and the Doctor :*

"The best Poor Law infirmary falls markedly below the standard of the London hospitals.

"It is, we think, impossible to avoid the conclusion that the Medical Branch of the Poor Law, now becoming an exceedingly costly service, is, at almost all points, in a far from satisfactory condition.

"In short, from the beginning to the end of a Poor Law expenditure of over £4,000,000 annually upon the sick, there is no thought of promoting medical science or medical education, practically no idea of preventing the spread of disease, and little consideration of how to prevent its recurrence in the individual[4]."

Lastly :

"To take the sick out of the Poor Law is, as we now see, the only way to put an end to what has inevitably a bad psychological reaction on personal character[5]."

The case is entirely different with regard to the public health service. Neither with the work of its officials, nor with the

---

[1] *Report of Poor Law Commission,* 1909, Q. 42509, par. 2.
[2] *The State and the Doctor,* p. 83.   [3] *Ibid.* p. 84.   [4] p. 128.   [5] p. 260.

numerous hospitals under its control, now spread all over the country, is there any fault to be found; but, surely, this result must be ascribed to the fact that here the State is attending mainly to its legitimate business, and is endeavouring not to *cure*, but to *prevent*, the spread of disease.

Under the crude and ill-considered clauses of the Insurance Act, however, it seems certain that an attempt is again to be made by the State at the treatment of tuberculosis, as well as of other diseases. Moreover, though it is somewhat difficult to find our way amongst the mazes of this Act, it seems probable that this treatment is to be carried out under very doubtful conditions.

In the first place, the ordinary treatment of a consumptive patient is to be conducted under the odious " contract " system, a system which has notoriously failed in the instances of Poor Law and of club practice. On this point I fully endorse what has been said by Dr Buttar in his recent letter to the *Morning Post*[1] :

" It is a pity that legislators who embark on revolutionary methods, such as the Insurance Act, do not, in the first place, get their minds thoroughly impressed with certain truths, such as the following. All contract practice is bad ; some contract practice is necessary ; therefore, keep your contract practice within the smallest limits possible ; and State service, though sometimes necessary, is not ideal. Therefore, foster rather the healthy growth of a natural system, that has developed in the course of ages, altering it gently only in such conditions as quite preclude its use."

Again, though an enormous sum has to be put aside for the establishment of sanatoriums and, perhaps, of dispensaries, these institutions will have to be mainly under the control of local Insurance Committees, who will be for the most part ignorant of medical science. The medical attendants of the institutions will be appointed by these authorities, and there will be no certainty that the doctors chosen will be competent to undertake the treatment of the multifarious forms of tuberculosis. Their chief recommendation to office will most likely be their acquaintance with some member or other of the local authority.

---

[1] September 16th, 1912.

Much of the money assigned for the purpose of the sanatoriums and of other objects will be wasted in various ways, especially in the erection of State buildings and in the carrying out of local " fads." We may be very sure that the local Medical Committees, appointed as a sop to Cerberus, will have very little voice in the matter. Hitherto our medical brethren seem to have hesitated to criticise this part of the chaotic scheme laid before them, partly, perhaps, because it is the most popular part of the Act, and partly because of the proverb against looking a gift horse in the mouth. Certainly the Royal College of Physicians expressly excluded sanatoriums from their purview when the bill was submitted to their consideration, and other associations of medical men have taken the same course. It is, however, very important that the subject should be seriously dealt with by medical critics before it is too late, and before the funds assigned for the purpose are in process of being squandered.

These illustrations may, perhaps, suffice to show that, in these several cases at least, the State has failed to take up efficiently the treatment of disease, especially of tuberculosis; and that, in the plans adumbrated by the Insurance Act, it is equally certain to fail.

In its ill-advised efforts the State is, in fact, departing from the wise counsels of that great political economist, John Stuart Mill, and is establishing permanent machinery to do work that could be better done in the future by voluntary agencies. Thus, in his monumental work on *Political Economy*[1], he says :

" A good Government will give all its aid in such shape as to encourage and nurture any rudiments it may find of a spirit of individual exertion."

And again :

" Government aid, when given merely in default of private enterprise, should be so given as to be, as far as possible, a course of education for the people in the art of accomplishing great objects by individual energy and voluntary co-operation[2]."

---

[1] Vol. II. p. 607.

[2] My friend, Mr J. W. Sharpe, has called my attention to the fact that Herbert Spencer is equally strong against the interference of the State with private concerns, especially by coercion. He quotes as follows from *Facts and Comments*, p. 24 (ed. 1902) : " The notion that a society is a manufacture, and not an evolution, vitiates

What, then, are the duties of the State in this regard ?   I venture to assert that they are summed up in the one word *prevention*.

Unquestionably, one of the most important duties of a State is the prevention of all disease that has been proved by medical science to be preventable. Happily, in this country this duty has not been neglected so far as most of the so-called zymotic diseases are concerned. Many hundred thousand lives have thus been saved by the energy of our public health services.

It is, however, only within recent years that tuberculosis has been fully recognised to be a preventable disease, and still more recently that it has come to rank as an infectious disease. It is true that in Italy and some other warm countries consumption has been reckonèd for many years an infectious disease ; but it was not until Villemin, in 1865, proved the fact by direct experiment, that it can be said to have fairly taken its place among the infectious disorders.

There are, however, several points in relation to the infectivity of tubercle which must be taken into account in considering the duties of the State in regard to its prevention. These points are, in brief :

(1)   First, the tenacity of life of the bacillus of tubercle, when fed with suitable material, and when left for long periods under what are known as unsanitary conditions.

(2)   Its resistance to ordinary disinfectants, to putrefaction, freezing and thawing, etc.

(3)   Its rapid loss of virulence under the influence of fresh air and sunlight.

(4)   The incubation period, and the temperature of growth, of the organism. It is no longer regarded as a pure parasite, existing only at the temperatures of the mammalian body. Many observers have now succeeded in growing it within wide ranges of temperature ; and I have myself grown it in the condensed vapour of human breath, and in that from ground air, at ordinary English spring and summer temperatures.

political thinking at large, leading to the belief that only by coercion can benefits be achieved. Is an evil shown ? then it must be suppressed by law. Is a good thing suggested ? then let it be compassed by an Act of Parliament."

(5) The infectivity of tuberculous dust, under differing circumstances of light and air.

(6) The association of the bacillus of tubercle with other organisms, such as the *tetragonus*, and various other cocci.

(7) The varying powers of resistance to infection offered by the human body. And, lastly,

(8) The researches as to the relations between bovine and human tuberculosis.

All these subjects have now been carefully studied, and will have to be taken into account in any concerted scheme for the prevention of the disease.

It must never be forgotten that infection by tubercle is conditional, and that the conditions under which it can take place are mainly three. They are : (1) The presence of a virulent form of the bacillus ; (2) a susceptible body to receive it ; and (3) such external circumstances as are favourable to infection.

Unless all these conditions are present it is unlikely that the disease will spread infectively through any community. Even when both the bacillus and a susceptible person are present, if the surrounding circumstances be such that the virulence of the microbe is destroyed before it can reach its victim, then no infection will take place.

There are, therefore, at least three distinct directions in which the State can employ its energies in the campaign against tuberculosis :

(1) It can take practical measures to abolish the bacillus.

(2) It can so improve the physical condition of the people as to diminish their susceptibility to the disease ; and

(3) Most important of all, the State can so amend its favourite haunts as to destroy its power for evil.

These, certainly, are no easy tasks to set before the State, but they are none of them impossible ; and the mere attempt to carry them out must end in the amelioration and lessening of the disease. We shall consider them in order.

1. *The Destruction of the Bacillus of Tubercle.*

It was perhaps natural that, immediately after Koch's discovery of the specific germ of tubercle, and after the proofs of its infectivity which he adduced, a popular cry should have been raised for stringent measures against infection. It was already known that the disease is very rarely congenital, and therefore it followed that nearly all of the 300,000 persons then suffering from it in England must have contracted the deadly complaint either directly from some other invalids, or indirectly by infection from tuberculous dust. It was logical to conclude that, if all these sufferers were treated like lepers and shut off from the rest of the community, and if other sources of infection such as tuberculous meat or milk were stopped, the disease would soon cease to exist, and the problem of its prevention would be solved.

There arose, accordingly, loud demands for compulsory notification of all cases of tuberculosis ; the penalisation of spitting ; gratuitous examination of sputum, etc., for the bacillus ; disinfection of the dwellings and clothing of tuberculous persons ; the provision of sanatoriums and of " homes for advanced cases," of dispensaries, and of colonies for quiescent cases. The State supervision of all cattle, and the formation of non-tuberculous herds, were also called for.

These measures are indeed, all of them, likely to be of great use, and will probably all have to be brought judiciously into action, sooner or later ; but the reformers have underrated the difficulties in the way of their task. Moreover, in some respects they go beyond, and in others they fall short of, the requirements of the case. Thus, if they were applied without discrimination to all cases of tuberculosis, they would inflict sore punishment upon many perfectly harmless individuals, and would brand them as if they were lepers. Dr Koch himself, in his last Nobel Lecture, sums up the case thus :

" Patients with closed tuberculosis are to be regarded as quite harmless. Even those who suffer from open tuberculosis are harmless so long as the tubercle bacilli expelled by them are prevented by cleanliness, airing, etc., from infecting. The patient becomes dangerous only when he is personally uncleanly, or becomes so helpless in consequence of the far-advanced disease that he can no longer see to the suitable removal of the sputa. For the healthy the danger of infection increases with the impossibility of avoiding the immediate neighbourhood of a dangerous patient—

that is, in densely inhabited rooms; and quite specially, if the latter are not only overcrowded but also badly ventilated and inadequately lighted."

The case could hardly be better put. Moreover, on the other hand, they would only remove some of the sources of infection, and would leave many others almost untouched. They would not cope with the dangers arising from the cases of incipient or of "walking" phthisis, nor from those who, if the measures were insisted upon, would undoubtedly hide the nature of their complaint.

They would also leave the most frequent sources of infection untouched. They would probably be of use to diminish the number of infecting persons, but they would do little to meet the many sources of ill health or of other diseases which prepare the way for the attack of the germs that had escaped the net, and which would continue to be only too abundant in unhealthy surroundings.

The State would therefore have to resort to further measures, and it should at least consider whether it were possible to do anything to diminish the second condition of infection—namely :

2. *The Susceptibility to Infection by Tubercle.*

It is not necessary to inflict upon you a discussion of the various forms of susceptibility to tubercle, whether inherited, constitutional, or acquired. It will be sufficient to point out that, though this condition of infection is difficult to remove entirely, it may be greatly mitigated.

With healthier homes, purer air in workshops and in places of public assembly, absence of microbic dusts, with better food and less alcoholic drinking—and all these reforms are attainable under wise governance—there would assuredly be fewer hosts for malignant guests in the shape of pathogenic microbes.

The measures that the State can take to mitigate the second condition of infection by tubercle are, therefore, identical with those required to meet the third—namely :

3. *The Removal of Unhealthy Surroundings.*

The State is fully competent to deal with this part of the subject ; and again its duty may be stated in one word—sanitation.

First, by the provision of healthy homes. Tuberculosis has been rightly termed a " house disease." I have myself shown in my paper on tuberculous infective areas, published in 1888 (see p. 176), that the disease clings to certain districts in Manchester and Salford, and even to certain houses; and similar observations have been made by Dr Niven and by Dr Flick of Philadelphia. Dr Flick says : " Of all diseases, tuberculosis, more than any other, is a house disease. It is implanted in the house, develops in the house, and it matures in the house."

Dr Koch, also, in his Nobel Lecture, remarks : " Tuberculosis has been frankly and justly called a dwelling disease."

Obviously, then, the first duty of the State is to see that the people are healthily housed ; and not only must the houses themselves be properly constructed, under stringent " building byelaws," but, by wise " town planning," by the destruction of neighbouring unsanitary property, by proper drainage and water supply, and by other measures, the air that circulates around these houses must be kept pure, and all such sunlight as this country affords must have full play upon them.

Fresh air and sunlight are the best disinfectants for the virus of tubercle ; and it is therefore the duty of the State to see that these important requisites are provided so far as may be possible. No one can, indeed, be compelled to open the windows of a dwelling; but householders can at least be tempted to do so by securing for them as far as possible the purity of the outside atmosphere.

The subject of ventilation as regards the prevention of tuberculosis is a very large one. It is probable that in confined air there exists some special nutriment which either serves to prolong the life of the bacillus or which increases its virulent properties, this special element being either the organic matter exhaled from human bodies, or the emanations from polluted ground air or from badly drained sub-soils.

It follows, therefore, that the State must not only make provision for cubic space in dwellings and for the admission of so many cubic feet of air to them, but that it must also see that this air is fairly pure, and that the ventilation shall sweep away " air-sewage " from these rooms and from all places where human and other beings congregate. Hence, also, in town planning, and in the reconstruction of unhealthy areas, free course must be given to the winds of heaven ; there must be no blind alleys or courts, and any pollution of the atmosphere must, as far as possible, be mitigated.

The ventilation not only of schools but of all places of public resort—such as churches, chapels, theatres, even public-houses, restaurants, and shops—must be placed under State control ; and all work-places and factories must be kept as clean as possible and well supplied with fresh air[1].

The height of buildings in the streets must be correlated with their width ; and ample " lung-space " must be provided in the shape of public parks and playgrounds.

The State will also be strictly within the scope of its legitimate action if it provides for the dangerous cases of open tuberculosis, if it subsidises homes for the dying and tuberculosis dispensaries, and if it assists the formation of herds of cattle, free from disease, as has been done in Denmark. But again I venture to protest against its meddling with the treatment of the disease in any of these cases.

In concluding this address, pray let me apologise for having once again repeated what has already been many times told. I am conscious that I have been preaching a very old sermon ; but, in mitigation of my offence, let me plead that my remarks have really been addressed to our rulers, that the State is well known to be very thick-headed, and that, as Jan Ridd said of the Devon folk, " At Oare, you must say a thing three times, very slowly, before it gets inside of the skull of the good man you are addressing."

---

[1] With reference to the last-mentioned places, I cannot help turning aside for a moment to complain of the recent retrograde step taken by the present Home Office in lowering the standard of ventilation of work-places and factories, which had been fixed by a former Committee of this Office. In place of restricting the amount of respiratory impurity, 9 vols. of CO_2 per 10,000 vols. of air, they now permit 11 vols. This is distinctly a retrograde step.

Chart II (a)

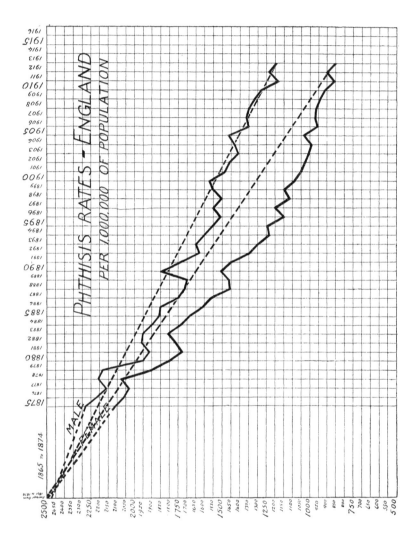

(7) THE NEED OF CO-ORDINATION OF ANTI-TUBERCULOSIS MEASURES

Paper read at the Fifth Annual Conference of the National Association for the Prevention of Consumption, August, 1913

THE charts show in graphic form the rise and fall of phthisis rates in England and Wales. Chart I (facing p. 1) gives the rate per ten thousand of persons since the beginning of the registration of the causes of death, by the late Sir W. Farr, in 1838. Chart II (a) (on opposite page) gives the rate per million for males and females separately since the year 1875; and at the beginning of the curves this chart gives also the average rates during the decade 1861–1870 inclusive.

In the year 1882 the nature of the true cause of the disease, the bacillus of tubercle, was discovered by the late Dr Robert Koch. Chart II (a), therefore, may be expected to point to the influence of this discovery and of the measures of repression which since then have been put into force to diminish the fatality of the disease.

First, one must note that all these sets of curves are, on the whole, on the down grade; that the female phthisis rate has been lowered from 2100 per million at the beginning of the period displayed in Chart II (a) to about 850 at the end. The male rate has also gone down, though at a slower pace, from about 2500 per million to nearly 1250. In other words, the former figures are about one third and the latter about one half of what they were fifty years before.

Perhaps I may be allowed incidentally to remark that, so far, the prophecy which I hazarded fourteen years ago, in 1899, seems likely to be fulfilled. I then said[1] : "When all our forces are brought fully into action, we may surely expect that at least as great a rate of decline will be continued, and, in that case, another thirty years should see its vanishing point."

In the same paper, however, I also said, "We can hardly doubt that the retreat will go on at an increasing speed"; but unfortunately that has not been the case; it is disappointing to see from

---

[1] "On the Prospect of Abolishing Tuberculosis," *Trans. Epid. Soc.* N.S. vol. XVIII. (See Paper 3, Sect. IV. in this volume.)

these charts that, in fact, the rate of diminution in the rates during the last twenty years has been somewhat less than it was formerly.

It may safely be asserted that no direct repressive measures against the disease had been taken until about twenty years ago. The steady improvement in the phthisis rate during the early portion of the period cannot therefore be ascribed to this influence. It can only have been due to general sanitary reforms and to a gradual rise in the resisting powers of the population.

This fact, together with the failure of frontal attacks upon the disease, brings us to various queries as to the best tactics for the completion of the campaign against the enemy.

(1) What were the chief measures that were so successful in controlling the disease in the earlier portions of the period in question ? I have already[1] given reasons for grouping these agencies under the heads of—(a) ventilation; (b) land drainage ; (c) the sanitary improvement of dwellings ; (d) the amelioration of social conditions ; (e) temperance.

(2) Why should the rate of diminution of the male deaths have so persistently lagged behind that of the females ? Is it not due to the fact that women have been " keepers at home," and have thus profited more from the improvement of their dwellings ; while the men herd together more in common lodging-houses, in public-houses, and in badly ventilated work-places, and everywhere spit about the floors of all these places ?

(3) Has there been any slackening in the zeal of sanitary reformers ? So far as regards medical officers of health and sanitary authorities, the answer to this question ought certainly to be in the negative ; but, owing to the greater attention now being paid by the Legislature to the provision of sanatoria, the use of various forms of tuberculin, the establishment of tubercle dispensaries, and other modes of *treating* the disease when established, the true object of the whole movement, namely, its *prevention*, is being neglected by the general public.

Are there not still whole areas of insanitary houses in most of our towns and villages where the disease still prevails three or four times as much as in the more healthy districts ?   And can we look with complacency on the incidence of phthisis upon those classes

---

[1] " On Phthisis Rates," *Trans. Epid. Soc.* N.S. vol. XXIV. (See Paper 5, Sect. IV. in this volume.)

of work-people employed in trades where the ventilation is insufficient ? And, in this regard, I would again call attention to the serious retrograde step taken last year by the Home Office, by which the standard of ventilation in certain work-places has been greatly lowered.

(4) Lastly, what tactics should be pursued in the further proceedings against the enemy ?

Without doubt, all measures for direct attacks upon the disease should be encouraged to the utmost. The various authorities concerned in the strife should persevere with the notification of the disease, the disinfection of infected places, the provision of places for the segregation of all cases of " open tuberculosis," and should take care that the purity of the milk and food supplies is secured.

We must not, however, rest satisfied with these " Continental " methods, but should also insist upon the carrying out of all those measures of sanitary reform which have already done so much to reduce the mortality from phthisis in this country.

To repeat what I have said before (in the paper already quoted) : " Much as has been accomplished, much more remains to be done in the way of opening up the blind streets and alleys in our large towns, the destruction of insanitary property, the building and proper management of healthy dwellings for the poor— not only in towns, but also in the country—and the preservation of as pure an atmosphere as possible.

" More persistent efforts will also have to be made to obtain herds of tubercle-free cattle throughout the country."

There still remain many of the adverse influences which we have seen to weigh so heavily, especially upon the male phthisis rates ; and all these will have to be tackled.

We must not rest satisfied with promoting only the frontal attacks upon the enemy ; it must also be taken on the flank and rear. All possible breeding places of the disease must be thoroughly cleared out ; the natural disinfectants, fresh air and sunlight, must be allowed free play ; the filthy habit of spitting must be put down with a strong hand ; and, finally, not only the homes, but all the places of work of artisans, and all their places of public resort, must be swept clear of "air-sewage," and a fit standard of ventilation and of purity and cleanliness must be enforced.

SECTION II. CONDITIONS OF INFECTION

(1) ON THE LIMITS OF INFECTION BY PHTHISIS

Public Health, *January*, 1895

THE agitation of the public mind at the present time on the subject of the infectiousness of tubercle, may justly be designated as a "scare." The dread of this occurrence is out of all proportion to the danger ; it goes far beyond what the facts of the case justify ; it is likely to cause grievous injustice to many poor invalids, and, in some cases, to endanger their prospects of cure.

The utterances and writings of not a few medical men tend to add to this distress of mind.

Leaflets and papers are issued describing consumption correctly enough as an "infectious disease," and giving truly excellent advice as to the disinfection of sputum, clothing, etc., but either altogether omitting to mention the limits of infectiveness, or relegating, to a short paragraph at the end of the document, the simple conditions of entire safety in proper sanitary surroundings.

I shall only cite two instances in proof of these statements.

1. From a memorandum issued by a Society of Medical Officers of Health under the following heads :

" (1) *Kind of disease.* It has been abundantly proved that ' phthisis ' or ' consumption ' is an infectious disease.

" (2) *Source of infection.* It does not appear that this disease is very, if at all, infectious through the breath of a patient ; but it is quite certain that it is infectious by means of the sputum (expectoration) which a sick person coughs up from his diseased lung.

" (3) *Infective material easily dealt with.* The means for preventing the spread of phthisis, therefore, from person to person, are made very simple by reason of the infective material being easily recognisable.

" (4) *Manner in which the disease is usually spread from*

person to person. The manner in which phthisis is usually spread from one person to another by means of the sputum is as follows :

"(*a*) A consumptive patient coughs up a quantity of sputum, in which are enormous numbers of the specific germs, *bacilli tuberculosis* ;

"(*b*) The sputum lodges where it is spat, and there dries ;

"(*c*) When dried, the sputum is usually pulverised and floats in the air as dust ;

"(*d*) The germs contained in the sputum, though dried, are still living, and able to infect the air in which they are suspended ;

"(*e*) The infected air when breathed is liable to cause phthisis. This is more particularly true of people who are already suffering from phthisis and whose recovery is thus prevented."

Then follow elaborate directions as to disinfection, food, etc., and as to cleanliness, ventilation, etc., but nothing is said about the security given by these means.

2. A paper by Dr Arnold Chaplin, " On the Necessity for placing Tubercular Phthisis under Control," contains the following suggestions : (1) That the Notification Act shall apply to phthisis, a course that, with careful limitations, I would myself cordially support. (2) The prevention of patients with actual phthisis, or indeed with strong predisposition, from marrying. (3) Prohibition of patients, with actual phthisis, from frequenting churches, theatres, railway carriages, tramcars, or any public places. (4) Disinfection of sputa, habitations, and all things coming in contact with phthisical patients. (5) Isolation of the consumptive.

Dr Chaplin indeed remarks that " It is doubtful if at any time such regulations could come into force." But he adds, " Once firmly impress upon the mind of the public that phthisis is dangerous, and to be treated with antiseptic precautions, then some definite project of isolation and notification may be considered."

As Dr H. Bennet has well said, if such recommendations as these were carried out, " social relations would be all but disorganised, a consumptive patient would be considered like a leper in olden days, one to be separated from his family, to be isolated, shut up. He would have to live months, nay years, in a tent. His clothes should be destroyed, and whether he dies or recovers, the house which he has inhabited should be burnt. It would perhaps be a charity to mankind to kill him at once, like an animal attacked with rinderpest; for, as the duration of the ordinary forms of phthisis may extend over years, during that period every time he breathed he would be filling the atmosphere with the germs of disease, wafted by the winds to be scattered far and near. Such is the logical sequel of the doctrine of the contagion of phthisis, carried to an extreme, as it is now being carried by many, especially in Germany and France.''

The result of such teaching as I have described is already becoming apparent in many directions. Persons affected with almost any chest disease find it difficult to obtain places as domestic servants. The close ties of family affection are not always strong enough to induce relatives of consumptives to undertake what is considered to be the dangerous duty of nursing them. The sites for consumption hospitals are becoming as difficult to find as those for fever hospitals, and utterly unfounded reports as to the spread of the disease by such institutions are recklessly made, even by medical officers of health.

It has become important, therefore, to ascertain the true state of the case, and to lay it judicially before the public.

The controversy as to the possibility of contracting consumption by contagion, is a very old one. It dates from the time of Galen, and even earlier. Great names are ranged on either side, and the fact that such men as Drs Andrew, Wilson Fox, and Theodore Williams, are ranged on one side, and Dr Weber and Dr Burney Yeo, on the other, ought to make us pause and hesitate before we dogmatise on the subject.

It is, however, impossible to avoid remarking in this, as in so many other controversies, that the combatants are often not meaning or talking of the same things, that they do not discriminate between *direct* and *indirect* infection, and that they frequently neglect to inquire as to the essential conditions of danger or safety. There are now few medical men who do not believe that a bacillus is the essential cause of phthisis, and that, as a rule, the organism enters the body from without, in the respired air, in food, or in drink; but there are many who do not sufficiently take into account the circumstances which alone can permit it to develop its virulent qualities.

In the words of the late Dr Addison, in reference to certain other infections, " they forget that one blade of the destroying shears may be forged at home, and without it the other cannot do its work." In truth, as I shall presently show, under a certain set of conditions, the infection of tubercle is one of the commonest events ; under another it is, in this climate, one of the very rarest.

Let us briefly review the history of the growth of the idea that consumption is communicable, and analyse the facts upon which it was originally founded.

The opinion that phthisis is an infectious disease, to be treated and to be rigorously dealt with as such, has been held for centuries in the South of Europe, notably in Spain and Italy, and it is quite possible that in these hot climates, the conditions of life may be especially favourable to the attack of the specific organism. But it is only quite recently that the idea has gained any vogue in this country, in France, or in Germany.

In 1859, indeed, Dr Gueneau de Mussy contributed a paper to *L'Union Médicale* (No. 138), in which he contended that phthisis is communicable by co-habitation, and that it is most frequently transmitted from husband to wife ; but he expressly repudiates the doctrine of Morgagni, who believed in the direct contagiousness of the disease. Dr William Budd also, in 1867[1], propounded the view that tubercle is a true zymotic disease, and that the tuberculous matter is itself (or includes), the specific morbific material, by which phthisis is propagated from one person to another; and that, by the destruction of this matter, on its issue from the body, seconded by good sanitary conditions, there is good reason to hope that we may rid ourselves of this fatal scourge.

It does not appear that this remarkable anticipation of recent doctrines met with any general assent at the time ; on the contrary several eminent physicians, amongst whom was Dr Wilks, attempted to controvert these views. Five years later Dr Weber's important paper " On the Communicability of Phthisis " attracted much more attention. It was not, however, until after Koch's great discovery of the essential organism of tubercle, that any

---

[1] *Lancet*, vol. II. p. 451.

idea of serious danger occurred to the medical mind. The report
of the Collective Investigation Committee of the British Medical
Association undoubtedly strengthened the feeling in favour of
Dr Budd's view, although, out of 1078 answers to the question,
" Is Phthisis Contagious ? " only 261 were affirmative, 778 were
negative, and 39 were doubtful. It is noticeable that all witnesses
to the case for contagion rely mainly upon the coincidence of
one or more cases of the disease, following co-habitation or attendance upon phthisical patients, and that, throughout the report,
little is said as to the surrounding conditions, which were really
in almost every instance the true sources of the infection. In
only 26 cases is the subject mentioned, but in one (No. 166)
Dr Dewar, of Arbroath, strikes what should have been the keynote
of the inquiry by remarking that, in all his cases " the patients
lived in small, confined houses, and slept in the ' box-beds ' in
use in Scotland." He adds, " During twenty-five years, I have
not seen one case of contagion in the airy houses of the well-to-do."

In a lecture " On the Limits of the Infectiveness of Tubercle,"
delivered in 1884, I ventured to point out other defects in the
record, and it is probable that even yet not much effect was
produced on the mind of the public. The most widespread
influence in the alarmist direction was really due to Dr Cornet.
He gave a detailed account of the fearful mortality from consumption amongst the nursing orders in Germany. His experience,
though it is given with a greater elaboration of detail, after all
only confirms that of many others, and notably of Luzuriaga, in
1787, and of Laennec, in 1820. But he followed up this inquiry
by an experimental research, as to the presence of actively virulent
bacilli in the dust derived from the rooms of persons affected with
phthisis. He succeeded in giving tuberculosis to a certain proportion of the animals inoculated with this dust, and although
this success does not measure the extent of danger to human
beings simply from inhalation, it shows that the bacillus will
survive for a certain time in the wards of hospitals, in hotel
bedrooms, and in the dwellings inhabited by these people.

But again I must point out that nothing is said as to the
conditions conducing to the continued vitality of the bacillus.
I have searched carefully through these documents, and little

or nothing is said on the subject. Hence these researches add nothing to the weight of the evidence, and do little more than emphasise our directions as to cleanliness and ventilation. Throughout the whole of the evidence hitherto adduced, therefore, there is to be noted the same defect, *hiatus valde deflendus*, an almost total lack of appreciation of the importance of the conditions favouring or attenuating the power of the bacillus for evil. And yet there are plenty of indications of the necessity for taking these circumstances into account in such an inquiry as this. Long before the discovery of the bacillus, and therefore before any measures of disinfection had been practised, the power of free ventilation to prevent the disease was fully recognised.

If the contagion theory were correct, hospitals for consumption should have been, at any rate in the past, centres and hotbeds of infection. But the universal testimony of the physicians to these institutions is that no such conveyance of the disease can be traced in any such institution. It would almost appear, from the statistics brought forward, that their wards were the safest places in which susceptible persons could take up their abode. I may say that my own personal experience, after fifteen years at the Manchester Hospital for Consumption, is entirely favourable to this view. In several instances patients, in whom the disease had become quiescent during their stay in hospital, remained as domestic servants for longer or shorter periods, in one or two cases for over a year, and yet no re-infection took place. Moreover, during the period mentioned, no case of phthisis appeared in any of the continually changing official population of the hospital.

On the other hand, it was a common and most disheartening experience to find that patients, who had been apparently cured in the institution, on their return to their probably infected houses, speedily developed fresh outbursts of the disease[1].

Again, the phthisis death rate in the army and navy, in public institutions, and in populations, before, compared with that after, the introduction of free ventilation into their habitations, proves the absolute necessity of taking this factor into account.

---

[1] See paper on "Re-infection in Phthisis," *Medical Chronicle*, October, 1892. (See Paper 5, Sect. III. in this volume.)

Without going any further, the statistics of Dr Cornet himself would be amply sufficient to support this contention.

It may be confidently affirmed, without fear of contradiction, from a broad survey of the facts, that, wherever plenty of nature's disinfectants, pure air, light, and dry and pure soil, are to be found, there consumption is rare; but wherever there is over-crowding, filth, and darkness, it breeds rapidly, and carries off large numbers.

It is constantly to be observed that the same races of men under one set of conditions escape its ravages almost entirely, and under another are seriously exposed to its attacks.

We are told by both Lombard and Hirsch that there is almost complete immunity from the disease in Nubia and Upper Egypt, in Asia Minor, Syria, Arabia, and Persia. Yet in Asia Minor it is often met with on the coast and in the principal towns. The Bedouins on the coast of the Red Sea, who exchange their tents for stone-built houses, suffer from consumption. In Syria it is met with at Aleppo, and in the Soudan at Khartoum. In Zanzibar it is said to be especially common among Arabian women of the higher class, owing to their greater seclusion. Whilst it is rare amongst the native Persians, who lead an almost open air life, it is more common amongst foreigners. In Algeria, whilst the nomad Arabs are free, amongst the captives many die from the disease ; and in Egypt, it is noted that whilst Syrians, Turks, Armenians, and Europeans seldom contract the complaint, Jews often become scrofulous, and frequently die of consumption.

Ruelhe[1] notes that Icelanders frequently contract the disease on removal to Denmark ; and so also do negroes who are brought from the interior to the coast or to Europe.

The wretched natives of Australia escape the disease almost entirely, but in the large towns of that continent it is as common as it is in Europe. The Highlanders, who inhabit well-built houses on the mainland of Scotland, are subject to the same fate as the other inhabitants; whilst the ill-fed, ill-clothed fishermen of St Kilda and the Hebrides, who are of the same race, hardly ever contract the disease. A striking case under this head is quoted by Dr H. Bennet, from Professor Hind. "Consumption,"

---

[1] Ziemsen, vol. v. p. 491.

he says, " is unknown amongst the natives of Labrador, whilst they remain in their own country. Here they live a kind of wild life in tents made of spruce branches, imperfectly lined with skins, and more or less open to the air. They are exposed to famine and all kinds of hardship, but when they come down the great river St Lawrence to take part in the fisheries, they occupy well-built houses, and being well paid, they live in comparative luxury ; and then many of them, in the course of a year or two, become consumptive, and thus miserably perish."

Again, nearer home we do not find that men who are much in the open air are especially prone to affections of the lungs. Soldiers on campaign, sailors, fishermen, hunters, gipsies, engine-drivers, coachmen, gardeners, agricultural labourers—none of these people suffer much from consumption, unless they are intemperate.

On the other hand, people who inhabit close, badly-ventilated, ill-lighted, badly-drained houses are peculiarly liable to the disease. We need not seek far for an explanation of these facts. They obviously point to some influence in or about the dwelling.

In a paper, read before the Epidemiological Society, in 1888, " On Tubercular Infective Areas " (see p. 176), I called attention to the existence in our large towns of centres of infection in the dirty, over-crowded, unventilated, and otherwise unsanitary courts and alleys of Manchester and Salford, and I put forward the hypothesis of the existence of specially infected areas, in which either polluted ground air, or an atmosphere reeking with organic matter, has given virulence to the organised germ of the disease, much in the same way as sewage or polluted water contributes to the conveyance of cholera or enteric fever.

These observations were supported by similar researches by Dr Tatham, of Manchester, and Dr Niven, then of Oldham.

In another paper, " On the Need of Special Measures for the Prevention of Consumption," read before the International Congress of Demography and Hygiene, in 1892[1], I adduced further reasons for this view, but suggested that the special nutriment, to be found in these houses, might merely serve to prolong the life of the bacillus, and thus increase the danger of infection. There are ample proofs in the researches of Koch, Bollinger,

---

[1] *Trans. of the Congress* p. 2741.

Galtier, and others, that the bacillus is very long-lived under some conditions, but, until lately, very few to show the reasons for the immunity of well-ventilated, well-lighted houses. The disinfecting power of natural agents seems to have been inadequately tested, except in the case of light by Koch; and these researches were chiefly carried out on pure cultivations, and not on dried and pulverised sputum.

In 1890, I made a communication to the Royal Society, "On Certain Conditions that modify the Virulence of the Bacillus of Tubercle[1]." In this paper, with the help of Prof. Dreschfeld, of the Owens College, I contrasted the behaviour of the bacillus in an unsanitary cottage in Ancoats, in a consumption hospital, and in a healthy, well-ventilated house. So far as these researches extended, they went to prove that fresh air and light, and a dry, sandy soil, have a distinct influence in arresting the virulence of the tubercle bacillus; that darkness somewhat interferes with this disinfectant action; but that mere exposure to such light as could be obtained in otherwise bad sanitary conditions does not destroy the virus.

In the present year, 1894, Prof. Delépine, of the Owens College, joined me in the work, and we carried the research a step further. We endeavoured amongst other objects, to determine how short a period of exposure to air and light would suffice to destroy the virulent action of the microbe. The results were communicated to the Royal Society in May last, and published in vol. LVI. of the *Proceedings* (page 51).

The experiments were made both with pure cultivations and with dried sputum, in some cases scraped and reduced to dust. Guinea-pigs were used for the inoculations. The experiments with the dried sputum are the most interesting, as they conform most closely with what would be met with in practice. The specimens were exposed for short periods only—two, three, and seven days—though control specimens were kept for long periods of time in darkness, and with very slight access of air. It was observed that, in all the specimens exposed in the dark, tuberculosis was the result even in free currents of air. The necessary minimum of such exposure to air, therefore, was not discovered,

---

[2] *Proc. R.S.* vol. XLIX. p. 66. (See Paper 4, Sect. III. in this volume.)

only three days being allowed to pass before the specimens were removed from the air current, but it was rendered evident that air alone somewhat attenuated the virus, even in the dark. On the other hand, all the specimens exposed to both air and light, even for two days only, and those exposed for one hour to sunshine, were found to have entirely lost their power for evil. Specimens of the same tuberculous dust gave tubercle to guinea-pigs after it had been kept in the dark, and with very little air, for thirty-five days.

It must be remembered that these tests were much more severe than would occur under ordinary circumstances. The animals employed were the most susceptible to the disease that could be found, and they took the virus through inoculation, and not merely by breathing; the usual safeguards against infection by the latter route, therefore, were entirely absent; and human beings might be expected to be much less vulnerable than guinea-pigs and rabbits.

It was doubtless important that these researches should be made, and that they should be repeated by others, for, if confirmed, they would explain the immunity from consumption of certain districts, and the infected character of others. I do not think, however, that they ought to be considered as indispensable. If men could have given its due weight to the strong circumstantial evidence that preceded the direct proof, they would have recognised long before this the limitations of the infectiveness of tubercle. The history of the disease, and its distribution throughout the world and throughout society, would have been quite sufficient to place them on the right track. In reality, the circumstantial evidence goes somewhat beyond the direct, for we can hardly suppose that, in the well-ventilated houses, there were no dark corners in which tuberculous dust had lodged for a longer or shorter time, and yet we can affirm that no infection took place.

The direct experiments show the probable mode in which the disinfection was accomplished; and they point out the line that should be taken in any measures having for their object the eradication of tubercle from our midst. In the words of the dying Goethe, " more light " is what we want, conjoined with more air, and greater cleanliness in our houses.

Let me not be misunderstood ; I do not wish to discourage any of the measures that have been proposed for the limitation of the disease, with the exception of the preposterous proposal for the entire segregation of all cases of the disease. By all means let us have notification of phthisis, directions for the disinfection and disposal of discharges from the body, and hospitals for the cure of the disease, and for the reception of the dying poor ; but in advocating these measures let us remember and guard against the inevitable effect upon the public mind of spreading these doctrines broadcast, unless they are accompanied by reassuring annotations as to the absolute security that is given by efficient ventilation by night and by day, by good drainage, and by an adequate supply of light.

Let us put our chief reliance upon, and all our energies into procuring, these essential requisites of all sanitation. Let us see to the thorough removal of " air-sewage," not only from living rooms, but also from the quarters of the working and the poor populations of our large towns.

Be strict as to the ventilation of all places of public assembly, their constant cleansing, and if necessary their disinfection ; and let the inspectors of markets, dairies, cowsheds, etc., be vigilant against the entrance of the disease by these channels.

It is mainly to measures such as these that is due the great diminution of the phthisis death-rate in the last thirty years.

A saving of over 1000 lives per million, or of about 30,000 persons in England and Wales, every year, from this cause alone, is certainly not owing to disinfection, but to general works of sanitary reform.

Surely it is within the province of medical officers of health, and in every way to the advantage of public health, to make these facts known, rather than to strike a note of alarm as to the contagiousness of phthisis that goes beyond the facts, and that may end in making the lot of many poor sufferers well-nigh unbearable.

Note.—I append a simple form of leaflet on the " Prevention of Consumption," issued by the Manchester and Salford Sanitary Association. It contains what is essential and yet is not alarmist in tone.

Prevention of Consumption.

It is now well known that consumption is often caused by the breathing of matter coughed up by consumptive persons, which, when it becomes dry, is blown about in the air as dust. This dust contains the poison which is the active cause of the disease ; if it is left in contact with any filth, or floating about in foul air, it is dangerous even to healthy persons, but it is especially hurtful to those with weak lungs, THOUGH IT SEEMS TO BE HARMLESS IN CLEAN, WELL-VENTILATED, WELL-DRAINED HOUSES.

It is therefore the duty of all persons suffering from this disease to take care that all expectorated matter is destroyed at once and not allowed to get dry and powdery, AND TO SEE THAT THEIR HOUSES ARE IN GOOD SANITARY CONDITION.

To ensure this being done, the following rules should be observed :

(1) All matter coughed up from the chest should either—

    (*a*) Be spat into the fire, or

    (*b*) Should be received in a vessel lined in such a way with a piece of paper, that the paper and its contents may be lifted out and burnt.

(2) Rags which can be burnt should be used instead of pocket handkerchiefs, and if a pocket handkerchief is used, it should be well boiled before the matter upon it has had time to become dry and powdery.

(3) The rooms and furniture used by persons suffering from advanced consumption should be frequently cleansed by washing with soap and water, and should also from time to time be thoroughly disinfected. All unnecessary bedhangings and curtains should be removed....

(4) As plenty of fresh air is absolutely necessary to persons suffering from or threatened by consumption, their houses should be kept clean, and thoroughly ventilated. If this is done it will greatly aid in the cure of the disease, and there will be no danger of contagion.

The windows, both of the living-rooms and bedrooms, should be kept open more or less, according to the weather, day and night, although direct draughts should be avoided.

If the clothing and bedding are sufficient, mere cold need not be feared ; but, if possible, a fire should be kept burning in the room to ventilate it.

THE CHIMNEY SHOULD NEVER BE BLOCKED UP.

(5) Consumptive persons, or persons threatened with consumption, should spend as much time as possible in the open air, and should keep away from close and crowded rooms, whether they be concert halls, meeting-houses, theatres, public-houses, or the like.

(2) THE SUSCEPTIBILITY OF TUBERCULOSIS UNDER DIFFERENT CONDITIONS

From THE PRACTITIONER *for* June, 1898

THE conscientious labours of the older writers have left very little to be done in the way of noting the incidence of tuberculosis upon the several classes of the population. Farr, Ancell, Wilson Fox, Walshe, and a host of Continental writers, have accumulated a mass of statistics on this point, which has been only slightly added to by more recent labourers in this field, and their conclusions from the facts thus collected have in the main been fully sustained.

Since Dr Koch's great discovery of the tubercle bacillus, however, it has become necessary to view all these researches in the light thus thrown upon the subject.

The subjects which now need to be regarded from the point of view of the new discoveries are : race, climate, local distribution of the disease, age, sex, heredity, and the nature and condition of soil.

Race.

No race of mankind can be said to be entirely exempt from the danger of contracting tuberculosis. Under certain conditions of environment, individuals of every race may contract the disease. Given a sufficient dose of actively virulent tubercle bacilli, and the possibility of contracting inflammatory affections of the lungs, no man can be considered safe from infection by this organism.

The experience of the most stalwart troops of the British Army in all climates of the world is sufficient to prove this statement.

The same races of men also, who, under one set of conditions, escape the ravages of phthisis almost entirely, under another are seriously exposed to its attacks. Thus the Bedouins on the coast of the Red Sea, who are usually exempt, yet suffer from consumption when they " exchange their tents for stone-built houses." In Algeria, the nomad Arabs are free from the disease, but amongst the captives many die from it. Again, the Highlanders, who inhabit well-built houses on the mainland of Scotland, are subject to the same fate as the other inhabitants ; but the ill-clothed, ill-fed fishermen of St Kilda and the Hebrides, who are of the same race, but who live much in the open air, hardly ever contract the disease.

Similar statements are made respecting the natives of Labrador, and other instances are given by Dr MacCormac, in his work *On the Breath Rebreathed*[1].

Ruelhe remarks that "Icelanders frequently contract the disease on removal to Denmark, and so also do negroes brought from the interior of Africa to the coast or to Europe."

There would be nothing surprising, however, in the discovery of a difference in the susceptibility of different races to infection by tubercle. Certain classes of animals, such as the carnivora—dogs, cats, Algerian rats—also sheep, goats, and horses, are usually refractory to infection by the specific bacillus of tubercle, whilst others, such as guinea-pigs and rabbits, are more susceptible. Yet Professor Delépine has shown that even the refractory animals may be made to contract tubercle.

Man is undoubtedly one of the more refractory animals, but it seems probable that some races, apart from the conditions of their surroundings and mode of life, are much more prone to tuberculosis than others. It has thus been especially noted that negroes and the native races of recently colonised places are peculiarly subject to the disease.

Hirsch tells us that "in Algiers, as in many other tropical or sub-tropical countries, it is the negro race that seems to be the most subject to the disease." In Senegambia the death-rate from phthisis among the French garrison, from 1862 to 1865, was 2·7 per 1000 of the total strength. In a battalion of natives numbering 450 men there were 23 deaths from consumption in fifteen years, giving a mortality of 3·4 per 1000 per year. Carbonell says : "La population noire du Sénégal est, comme partout ailleurs, très sujette à la phthisie."

Hottentot soldiers at the Cape suffer more from pulmonary phthisis than white soldiers ; so, too, at Sierra Leone, blacks

---

[1] p. 47.

furnish a larger quota of chest disease than white soldiers, in the ratio of 6·4 to 4·9 per 1000 (Boudin).

The Army Medical Report for 1859 states that, while not a single white soldier was admitted for tuberculous disease in Jamaica, the phthisical deaths among the negroes stood at 6·87 per 1000 of the strength.

Dr Andrew has, however, called attention to the interesting fact that this race may escape phthisis in one country and yet suffer from it in another. Thus the West Indian negro, not specially prone to it in his native land, becomes so when transferred to the Gold Coast, and this, too, although his near relatives there escape almost entirely. Dr Andrew remarks : " Here we have two very closely allied races living together, and yet the new comers suffer excessively from a disease to which they are at least as much exposed in their own country as the natives of the Gold Coast, who comparatively escape it, are in theirs." Under these circumstances, he thinks that the theory of race, and that of inoculation, are alike insufficient, and he suggests that there may be some modification of the bacillus itself.

With regard to the susceptibility of native races, Hirsch remarks that consumption is prevalent to a most disastrous extent among the native races of the Southern Pacific.

In New Caledonia the death-rate from consumption among the Kanakas is estimated at two-fifths of the mortality from all causes.

In New Zealand phthisis has made frightful ravages among the Maoris, and has become one of the chief causes of the gradual extinction of that race. In North Greenland the disease is one of the commonest causes of death, and it is common in Newfoundand, New Brunswick, and Canada—in the last, particularly among the native Indians.

It has been suggested by Mr Archdall Reid, in a work on the *Present Evolution of Man*, that in the older countries, where tuberculosis has been endemic for many generations, a certain tolerance of, or power of resistance to, the microbe has been acquired—a power due to " the accumulation of inborn variations " —and that they thus escape the full influence of the disease. Native races have not yet acquired this protective power.

Climate and Locality.

Not only is tuberculosis a disease of all races, it is also a disease of all countries and of all climates.

It is sufficient to glance at Hirsch's tables of the comparative mortality from consumption to see that all inhabited parts of the earth's surface are liable to the disease. He says : " It extends over every part of the habitable globe. It may be designated an ubiquitous disease in the strictest meaning of the term."

When we have taken a complete survey of the distribution of phthisis over the globe, we cannot, in fact, doubt that circumstances of climate are, on the whole, of very subordinate importance.

" The disease occurs, *caeteris paribus*, in all geographical zones with uniform frequency. Equatorial and sub-tropical regions are visited with consumption not less than countries with a temperate or an arctic climate. The differences that come out on comparing the amount of the malady in the several parts of a given zone are of the same kind as in all other zones. In many regions the number of cases has gone up considerably without any corresponding changes of climate, but under circumstances of quite another order."

In Dr Lombard's coloured maps of the distribution of phthisis, the only portions of the earth's surface from which the colour is entirely absent are the Arctic and Sub-Arctic regions, deserts, and high ranges of mountains, and it is precisely in those parts that human beings are fewest and most sparsely scattered over the ground.

In all the capitals of countries, and in the chief cities of Europe, Asia, Africa, and America, there is but little difference in the phthisis rate, and what differences there are cannot be accounted for by difference of climate.

TABLE I.—*Proportion of deaths from consumption to* 1000 *deaths at :*

London	..	..	..	121	Rome	..	..	..	114
Paris	..	..	..	143	Milan	..	..	..	132
Brussels	..	..	..	163	Lisbon	..	..	..	115
Vienna	..	..	..	208	Athens	..	..	..	183
Berlin	..	..	..	109	New York	..	..	167
Stockholm	..	..	160	Rio de Janeiro	..	..	186
Christiania	..	..	172	Lima	..	..	..	171
St Petersburg	..	..	151				(*Lombard.*)

In the light of our present knowledge of the essential cause of phthisis there is nothing surprising in our thus finding the disease wherever human beings are gathered together. The chief source of the organism which provokes the malady is the human race itself, and hence, unless there are adverse conditions, it might be expected to follow mankind in its distribution over the surface of the globe.

It must also be conceded that the other conditions of life under which people live are of much greater importance than the mere question of climate. The extreme variations of the disease in places geographically close together are so great and so frequent in most countries that they could not be due merely to differences of climate.

The fact is apparent at once upon glancing at any map of the distribution of phthisis—Dr Haviland's respecting England and Wales, Boudin's of France, and others of Norway and other countries.

But we may come to closer quarters still, and may take the areas of counties instead of countries, and note the variations of the phthisis rates within them.

The following table shows some of these variations in different parts of England, and care has been taken to note the presence of large hospitals, whose returns might vitiate our results.

TABLE II.—*Variations in the consumption rate, at ages 15–55, per* 100,000 *living at those ages* (*males*).

Counties	Towns	Highest	Lowest
Surrey . . .	{ Guildford	526	—
	{ Farnham	—	242
Sussex	{ Hastings	(H)643	—
	{ Battle	—	180
Oxford	{ Headington	(H)566	—
	{ Banbury	—	241
Cambridge ..	{ Whittlesea	469	—
	{ Wisbech	—	230
Norfolk	{ Walsingham	439	—
	{ Flegg	—	257
Wilts	{ Salisbury	438	—
	{ Mere	—	201
Cornwall ...	{ Redruth	461	—
	{ Launceston	—	223
Lincoln	{ Spilsby	361	—
	{ Caistor	—	205
Lancashire ..	{ Liverpool	(H)602	—
	{ Wigan	—	249
York	{ Reeth	589	—
	{ Settle	—	253

It will be noted that in most of the counties represented in this table the difference between the highest and lowest returns is more than 50 per cent. of the highest, and in some of them the highest reading is more than three times that of the lowest.

The same variation is to be found in other parts of the United Kingdom. Thus, in Scotland, consumption is almost unknown in the Western Hebrides ; but in towns on the west of the mainland, with very similar climate and a similar race of people, it is very common. In Ireland, again, the rate of mortality from the disease, per 100,000 of the population, in the ten years 1865–1874, was, in the eastern division, 259, in the western, 95. Similar variations are to be observed in other parts of the world.

Such facts as these might well lead us to the conclusion that mere locality and climate are absolutely of no importance, either in the prevention or the cure of tubercular disease ; but I am inclined to believe that we should be wrong in so deciding—at any rate, so far as locality is concerned.

There can be no doubt that circumstances—such as occupation, dwelling, the respiration of pure or foul air, liability to catarrhal affections, etc.—are of much greater importance than mere climate, and that they often determine the question of the infection of otherwise healthy persons ; but, when we take all these circumstances into consideration, it is still possible to find that certain climates and certain localities are less likely than others to promote the onset of the disease.

The natural history of the bacillus of tubercle, in fact, points out the places where the disease is likely to be most rife, and also those in which it is least likely to prevail.

The bacillus is best cultivated in a warm atmosphere, well charged with moisture, and containing plenty of nitrogenous organic impurity. I have myself found admirable media for its cultivation in wall-paper saturated with organic vapours from the breath and from ground air, and have ascertained that it is possible to grow it on these media at a temperature of about 60° to 70° Fahr., though it flourished more vigorously at higher temperatures of about 98°.

Now, when we turn to the statistics of Hirsch and Lombard, we find that it is the hot, damp climates of the world that are most exposed to the ravages of the more acute forms of phthisis.

There is ample proof of the frequency and special malignancy of the disease on the coasts of continents, and on islands placed within the tropics, and in other hot, damp, impure atmospheres.

It is common on both the east and west coasts of Mexico, on the coasts of Yucatan, Nicaragua, and Panama, though rare on the highlands in the interior of these countries ; and the disease is equally common and pernicious on the coasts and plains of Guiana, whilst it is almost unknown among the natives inhabiting the mountainous part of the country. It is also very frequent in all the islands of the West Indies, in Ceylon, and in the warmer regions of the Pacific.

It is increasingly prevalent in the coast districts of Chili, Peru, and Ecuador. " It is met with not uncommonly also among the deep valleys of the Andes, with a warm and moist climate, and in the forest region of Peru, even at elevations of 500 metres ; but the high plateaux are almost entirely free from it."

On the other hand, very dry climates are comparatively immune. In the inland districts of Lower Egypt and the valley of the Nile, phthisis, according to all observers, is very uncommon ; and in India " the localities specially distinguished by dryness of climate and uniformity of temperature, be they on the plains or among the hills, are least affected by phthisis."

The immunity from consumption of the three classes of districts which have already been mentioned in that regard—viz. deserts, Arctic regions, and mountain plateaux—may be, to some extent, due to their sparse population ; but it must be pointed out that they also, as a rule, have very dry atmospheres, and that the two last named seldom offer to the bacillus the encouragement of warmth and organic impurity.

It is especially interesting to speculate as to the causes of the antagonism of cold climates to consumption.

It is probable that cold hinders the growth of the bacillus outside the body, and thus tends to prevent both infection and re-infection of susceptible persons, as this infection certainly proceeds most frequently from virulent tuberculous dust from the walls and floors of insanitary dwellings. But we may surmise that the lower amount of humidity in the atmosphere of cold regions has also something to do with the result. Cold air has a much smaller capacity for moisture than warm air. It may thus be less capable of sustaining the life of the microscopic organisms which are the exciting causes of consumption; or, again, it is possible that there are smaller quantities of organically charged vapours arising from the ground, frozen as it is for so large a portion of the year. In a frosty air also the condensing moisture may entangle the organisms in the meshes of the frozen vapour, and may carry them down out of harm's way.

It must be again remarked, however, that there is no complete immunity from phthisis even in these favoured regions; it is quite possible to live in cold climates under conditions that will override all these opposing influences. It has been stated, for instance, that Iceland is almost free from phthisis, and that the Esquimaux do not suffer from it; but recent reports contradict both these assertions. In Greenland phthisis is one of the commonest causes of death, and similar reports come from New Archangel and Alaska.

In Canada also, at one time, soldiers sent to that station died of consumption at three times the rate of the ordinary civil population in England in healthy districts.

Somewhat similar remarks apply to the causes of the comparative immunity of mountain regions and elevated table-lands.

As to the fact itself there can be little doubt. In Lombard's map of the distribution of the disease, all the great mountain ranges are left blank—the Dovrefeld, the Ural Mountains, the Alps and Carpathians, the Apennines, the sierras of Spain, the Hartz, the Grampians of Scotland; in Asia, the high plateaux of Armenia and Persia, the Himalayas, and the chief mountain regions of China; the table-lands of Abyssinia and of Mexico, of Quito and the Andes.

Perhaps the greater degree of cold in these elevated regions may have something to do with this absence of disease; but it is probable that the less density of the population of these parts of the world is mainly instrumental in preventing pollution of the atmosphere with the bacillus and its favourite cultivating medium, organically charged vapour.

It is notorious that mountain and sea air are much freer from all kinds of organisms than the air of plains at a lower level.

Is it not likely also that the bracing, vivifying influence of such air may greatly strengthen the powers of the human frame to resist the inroads of the disease ?

Influence of Locality.

The causes of the influence of locality in determining the incidence of tubercular disease have also to be sought, and, as in the case of climate, they are intimately bound up with the habits and surroundings of the population.

Most of the differences in the phthisis rates of localities are due to the greater or less healthiness of their occupations, to the amount of air space in their workshops, the cleanliness or otherwise of their surroundings, the nature of the dusts to which their work gives rise.   But another, and perhaps a still more important, factor in the production of phthisis is the existence in certain localities of infected houses or even of infected areas.

It is now certain that the tubercle bacillus can not only exist for long periods of time, but even grow and flourish, in badly ventilated houses, built upon soil contaminated with organic matter, the vapour from which, if it is suffered to penetrate into the house, is one of the best cultivating fluids for this organism.

I have elsewhere called attention to the existence of these areas and of infected houses, and the observations have been confirmed by others—notably, by Dr Niven, of Manchester, and by Dr Flick, of Philadelphia.   These reports, which are further borne out by many of the returns made to the Collective Investigation Committee of the British Medical Association, afford ample proof of the potency of this cause for the spread of tubercular disease.

The researches which I have myself made as to the readiness with which the bacillus may be cultivated on wall-paper, saturated with impure aqueous vapours, may also be taken into account as showing the mode in which these insanitary houses may become infected.

There is, however, another circumstance more directly connected with locality, which must next be passed in review, and that is the influence of the underlying foundation soil and subsoil of dwellings.

Influence of soil.

Consumption is undoubtedly fostered by dampness in the subsoil of dwellings. In the year 1862 Dr Bowditch, of Massachusetts, made an elaborate inquiry into this subject, and came to the following conclusions :

(1) That a residence on or near a damp soil, whether that dampness is inherent in the soil itself or caused by percolation from adjacent ponds, from marshes or springy soils, is one of the primal causes of consumption in Massachusetts, probably in New England, and possibly in other portions of the globe.

(2) Consumption can be checked in its career, and possibly, nay probably, prevented by attention to this law.

Shortly afterwards, Dr Buchanan, then chief medical officer to the Local Government Board, came to much the same conclusions as the result of an elaborate research. These conclusions are worthy of being quoted *in extenso*. They were :

(1) Within the counties of Surrey, Kent, and Sussex there is, broadly speaking, less phthisis among populations living on pervious soils than among populations living on impervious soils.

(2) Within the same counties there is less phthisis among populations living on high-lying pervious soils than among populations living on low-lying pervious soils.

(3) Within the same counties there is less phthisis among populations living on sloping impervious soils than among populations living on flat impervious soils.

(4) The connection between soil and phthisis has been established in this inquiry (*a*) by the existence of general agreement in phthisis mortality between districts that have common geological and topographical features of a nature to affect the water-holding quality of the soil ; (*b*) by the existence of general disagreement between districts that are differently circumstanced in regard to such features ; and (*c*) by the discovery of pretty

regular concomitancy in the fluctuations of the two conditions, from much phthisis with much wetness of soil to little phthisis with little wetness of soil. But the connection between wet and phthisis came out last year in another way, which must here be recalled—(*d*) by the observation that phthisis had been greatly reduced in towns where the water of the soil had been artificially removed, and that it had not been reduced in other towns where the soil had not been dried.

(5) The whole of the foregoing conclusions combine into one—which may now be affirmed generally, and not only of particular districts—that " wetness of soil is a cause of phthisis to the population living upon it."

(6) No other circumstance can be detected, after careful consideration of the materials accumulated during this year, that coincides on any large scale with the greater or less prevalence of phthisis, except the one condition of soil.

Good drainage also has been found to diminish the prevalence of the disorder by as much as 50 per cent.

These results have since been confirmed by Dr Haviland and by the Registrar-General of Scotland. In the conclusions drawn from his map of the distribution of phthisis in England and Wales, Dr Haviland says : " Damp, clayey soil, whether belonging to the wealden, oolitic, or cretaceous formation, is coincident with a high mortality " ; and the Registrar-General, in his seventh report, remarks that " the towns, villages, hamlets, or houses which were situated at or near undrained localities, or were on heavy, impermeable soils, or on low-lying ground, and whose sites were consequently kept damp, had a very much larger number and proportion of cases of consumption than towns, villages, hamlets, or houses which were situated on dry or rocky ground, or on light, porous soils, where the redundant moisture easily escaped."

I have myself made an inquiry into this subject, the details of which are given in the Weber-Parkes Prize Essay for 1897, and which goes even further than those already cited—a contrast between two populations, one on clay lands, the other on a hill of sand. The results were derived from two series of mortality returns, one for the nine years 1875–84, the other for the succeeding nine years. Of the first group, twenty-two deaths were from phthisis, but eleven of them took place on certain low-lying clay lands which surrounded a hill of sand, and nine of the remainder were found by inquiry to have contracted the disease before coming to the place. This left only two to be accounted for. One of them was a gentleman who spent the greater part of his time in a neighbouring town, where he had frequently to attend crowded evening meetings ; the other was a merchant's clerk who went to town at eight every morning, and did not return till seven p.m. No woman or child died of the complaint. The disease, therefore, did not originate in any of the stationary population resident, during the nine years, upon the sandy portions of the district.

The results obtained in the second group were strikingly like those just given. Again the total for the nine years was twenty-two deaths from phthisis, and of these, nine were on the clay lands, thirteen on the higher ground—but seven of these were ascertained to have been imported. It may be remarked, also, that the population of the higher ground was five times as numerous as that on the low ground.

It is evident from these facts that there is a close relationship between the condition of the soil and consumption, and, although an attempt has been made to produce some counter evidence, it has not been sufficient to invalidate this conclusion. Thus the assumption of Boudin and others that a malarious soil is antagonistic to consumption has not been borne out by facts ; and certain instances of free drainage of the soil, without any corresponding diminution in the rate of mortality from the disease, have been shown to be due to the imperfect drying of the soil resulting therefrom.

But it is yet not clear how a damp subsoil can increase the tendency to phthisis. It has been supposed by some authorities that as a cold, damp soil tends to predispose to catarrhal affections, these diseases may so injure the lungs as to leave them more disposed to tubercular deposits. It is possible that there may be something in this hypothesis ; but there is certainly no definite relation between phthisis and other respiratory diseases. Thus at Birmingham, Macclesfield, and Brighton, whilst the phthisis rates are high, the deaths from other diseases of the respiratory organs are comparatively few. At Pickering, in Yorkshire, again, the phthisis rate is one of the lowest in the kingdom, yet the other diseases of the lungs are nearly as common as they are at Birmingham.

Such statistics as these are not, however, of much use in a question of this kind. It is well known that simple catarrhal affections of the lungs and chronic bronchitis rather diminish than increase the tendency to consumption, and hence a set of figures such as these, all lumped together, can give but little information of any value.

If it were possible to ascertain that there was a larger proportion of destructive inflammations—such as broncho-pneumonia, for instance—at Birmingham than at Pickering—a very likely event—it might be possible to account for the excess of phthisis in the former place, and thus for the discrepancy. In the existing condition of the Registrar-General's returns this is not now possible.

There is another, perhaps still more probable, explanation of the influence of soil in the greater or less proportion of impure aqueous vapours from the ground air in wet or dry soils respectively.

In the research[1] already alluded to, published in the Weber-Parkes Prize Essay for 1897, I have been able to show that these vapours when condensed afford an admirable cultivation fluid for the bacillus of tubercle, even at ordinary temperatures, and it can now hardly be doubted that this fluid is an important means of keeping alive and even enhancing the virulence of the organism in tubercle-infected houses. It is true that little difference in this respect was to be discovered between the vapours from pure and from impure subsoils; but it may reasonably be concluded that the air of houses on well-drained soils will be less likely to allow condensation of the vapour to take place on the walls or floors, than would be the case in houses less perfectly protected from the damp.

Probably both the influences that have been mentioned are usually at work to enhance the tendency of the disease to become endemic.

[1] See p. 159.

The Influence of Sex and Age.

These two subjects cannot well be considered separately. The incidence of tuberculosis upon the sexes is, to a great extent, determined by the occupation of the individual and the age at which it is carried on.

If we were to accept the returns of hospitals for consumption as truly representative, it would appear that men are greatly more liable than women to the disease. Thus, at Brompton Hospital, Dr C. T. Williams records that, out of 1000 cases, 625 were males, 375 females; and this accords with Dr James Pollock's experience, as among his out-patients 60·75 per cent. were males and 39·25 females.

In Dr Austin Flint's practice there was a still larger difference. Out of 669 cases in private practice, 321 were males, only 127 females; in hospital practice the number of male cases was 187, of female cases 37. (There is some discrepancy here.)

These results of hospital practice, however, must be due to some social cause, such as the inability of women to leave their homes in order to attend the hospitals. When the whole of the population of England and Wales is taken there is no such great discrepancy. Dr W. Ogle, in a letter to Dr Wilson Fox, published in his treatise on *Diseases of the Lungs*, points out that " there is practically no difference between the two sexes in their respective liability to death from phthisis. The mean annual mortality of males on an average of thirty years from this cause is 2418, and of females, 2428 per million living."

When these figures are corrected for age distribution there is a slight excess of males, the numbers being for them 2427, and for females, 2393.

The latest returns of the Registrar-General show that this difference is now greater, since the diminution in the female phthisis rate in the last decade is more considerable than in that of males. From 1881 to 1890 the numbers are : females 1609, males 1847 per million living.

How completely these respective phthisis rates are governed by other circumstances than that of sex is shown by the following table, which I drew up for the Milroy Lectures of 1890 :

TABLE III.—*Annual average proportion of deaths from consumption between the ages fifteen and fifty-five per* 100,000 *persons living at those ages between the years* 1861–1870.

Towns	Males	Females	Differences
Cambridge	570	395	−175
Whitechapel ...	560	430	−130
Bath	540	255	−285
Greenwich	525	375	−150
Brighton.......	520	345	−175
Southampton...	500	385	−115
Birmingham ...	475	345	−130
Newcastle......	470	395	− 75
Salisbury	440	305	−135
Sedbergh	365	615	+250
Congleton	360	595	+235
Bootle	225	555	+330
Leek	355	525	+170
Belper	275	455	+180
Buckingham ...	275	455	+180
Sevenoaks	290	455	+165
Alston	285	425	+140
Camelford	230	295	+ 65
Battle	180	365	+185
Pickering	160	315	+155
Billesdon	120	265	+145

The differences between these figures, concerning two groups, male and female, of the population of the same places, constitute the main points of my argument.

The influence of social condition and of occupation upon males and females respectively may be clearly discerned from this table; and although there is no distinct statistical evidence relating to female occupational mortality to be found in Dr Tatham's recent Supplement to the Fifty-fifth Annual Report of the Registrar-General, his table (V.), p. 161, shows the enormous influence of habits and occupation upon males. In this table, under the head of Phthisis, the " comparative mortality figure " for inn and hotel servants (London) is 607, that for coal-miners (Derbyshire and Nottinghamshire) is 69, and that for clergymen is 67, not much more than one-tenth of the first number.

We can hardly fail here to see the terrible influence of excessive drinking and of impure surroundings.

Yet, in spite of the overpowering influence of occupation and other conditions, there are some traces to be found of a true sexual susceptibility to tuberculosis.

In the letter from Dr W. Ogle, just quoted (p. 103), there is a suggestive table (D) which may here be given.

TABLE D.—*Mean annual mortality, 1861–80, per million living of children in each year of the first quinquennium of life from phthisis, hydrocephalus, and other tuberculous affections, male and female.*

	Under 1	1	2	3	4	All under 5 years
Phthisis :						
Males	1589	1341	634	394	339	880
Females ..	706	1295	655	409	360	842
Hydrocephalus :						
Males	4720	3851	1539	895	660	2399
Females ..	3167	2634	1178	733	552	1693
Other tubercular affections :						
Males	6553	3723	1256	571	369	2604
Females ..	5372	3370	1142	517	341	2231

It is evident from these figures that there is some special proclivity towards phthisis in the male infant. The male death-rate from phthisis in the first year of life is more than twice as high as the female rate; in the second year it is also the higher, but only to the extent of about 3½ per cent.; but in the third, fourth, and fifth years of life the female rate is slightly the higher.

This extra liability of the older females to phthisis continues till somewhere about thirty-five years of age, the maximum of excess being in the ten to twenty years of age period, when the excess reaches 50 per cent.; after this age the male rate is constantly, and generally considerably, in excess.

A similar excess is to be noticed in the rates of mortality of males from other tubercular diseases than phthisis, with this difference—that the male shows an increased tendency to these diseases almost throughout life.

We may perhaps conclude from these figures either that the male child is more susceptible to the tubercular virus, or else that his system resents its intrusion more intensely than that of the female.

Probably both these influences may be at work to produce the result.

Age.

It is well known that phthisis is a disease mainly of youth and middle age, the other tubercular diseases chiefly preferring to attack the young, under five years of age.

Quite the largest number of deaths from consumption take place between the ages twenty-five to thirty-five, and in the decade 1881–90 118,508 persons died of this disease at those ages out of 307,550 total deaths ; in other words, nearly half the deaths at this age were due to phthisis. But no age in either sex is entirely exempt from tubercular disease. It is true that congenital tuberculosis is extremely rare—so rare that Prof. Peters declares that " on ne naît pas tuberculeux mais tuberculisable," and Böllinger that " die sogenannte congenitale Tuberculose so gut wie auszuschliessen ist "—but several cases are reported in Verneuil's *Études sur la Tuberculose* and, as we have seen, it occurs with some frequency in the first years of life.

It also may occur at very advanced ages. Dr W. Ogle gives the phthisis rate per million at seventy-five and upwards as over 500 ; Sir Robert Christison found cavities in the lung of a man dying aged ninety-three, and Laennec met with it at the age of ninety-nine.

The Influence of Heredity.

The question of the influence of heredity in determining the incidence of tuberculosis has been discussed from time immemorial, and the exact nature of this influence must still be regarded as open to argument.

There are at least three modes in which tubercle may be regarded as hereditary : (1) The direct infection of a child with the disease in an active state before birth. (2) The congenital implantation of the organism, or of its spores, which may remain for a period latent in the system. (3) The transmission of organs, or of a bodily constitution, peculiarly open to attack by the bacillus—in other words, of an undue vulnerability of the system.

It is possible that any one or all of these circumstances may occur.

(1) We occasionally see cases of undoubted congenital tuberculosis, and the researches of Landouzy and Martin, of Lannelongue and of Niepce, already alluded to, show clearly the possibility of this event.

The first-named authors show[1] the tuberculising power of the seminal fluid of tuberculous guinea pigs. Niepce found bacilli in the semen of tuberculous individuals, though it is difficult to see how these could run the gauntlet through the placenta. Lannelongue, however, declares[2] in favour of the doctrine of the intra-uterine infection of the foetus, and he cites in support the aforesaid researches, and also the observations of Demme, who found in two infants, one of whom died on the twenty-first day after birth, an intestinal tuberculosis, and in the other, at the twenty-ninth day, a pulmonary tuberculosis with an advanced cavity in the lung[3].

These positive facts must be opposed to the negative experience of Leudet, who had never seen a case of foetal or congenital tuberculosis, whether hereditary or acquired, and to the observations of Vallin and of Straus, who regard the possibility of congenital tuberculosis, either in human beings or in calves, as entirely " negligible."

We may fairly conclude from this controversy that congenital tuberculosis is at least a rare disease, and that it cannot account for more than a very small proportion of the cases of alleged hereditary transmission of the disease.

(2) *Hereditary Transmission of Latent Germs of Tubercle.* This subject must be distinguished from that of the occurrence of cases of insidious inroads of tubercle without active symptoms, and also of cases of quiescence of tubercular deposits during long periods of time. These cases have been described as " latent," but they are not necessarily connected with heredity. What is now meant is the supposed transmission of germs which may

---

[1] *Études sur la Tuberculose*, pp. 59–67.

[2] *Op. cit.* p. 97.

[3] A number of references to cases of supposed congenital tuberculosis are given by Dr Wilson Fox (*Diseases of the Lungs*, p. 534, footnote 2.)

remain latent throughout childhood, adolescence, or even through the whole life.

Lannelongue and Baumgarten account for the rarity of infantile tuberculosis by supposing that the foetal tissues resist the action of the inherited germs ; and Baumgarten goes still further, and asserts that " tuberculosis may remain latent, under certain circumstances, during the whole of life without interfering with living functions in any observable degree." Nay, more : he believes that it may pass through a generation, and be transferred from grandparents to grandchildren. He places it in the same category with syphilis and leprosy, and ascribes the greater part of the tuberculosis in the world to this hereditary descent. He defends this thesis by an appeal to the cases and experiments already alluded to ; and he cites in its favour his own researches and those of Marchand, of Böllinger, and other pathologists, though, as we have seen, Böllinger is certainly not on his side.

I hardly think it necessary seriously to discuss this theory : there is no proof that the virulence of the bacillus can remain latent for more than a few months, the heredity of leprosy is still unproved, and the analogy of syphilis to tuberculosis is not yet made out. Dr Baumgarten also surely underestimates the great weight of the evidence that connects phthisis with the inhalation of impure air and with indoor occupations. We may, I think, reject this hypothesis as untenable.

(3) *The Hereditary Transmission of a Susceptible Consti-tution.* There is much more to be said in favour of the view that parents may transmit to their offspring a peculiarly vulnerable constitution.

It has been noticed since the days of Galen and Aretaeus that there is often a peculiar shape of the thorax in phthisical persons. This form of chest has been ascribed to smallness of the lungs and to undue rigidity of the bones. According to Sir W. Jenner, the essential feature is " the straightening of the upper ribs, with widening of their intercostal spaces, and undue obliquity of the lower ribs, whose intercostal spaces are narrowed." The thorax is thus flattened in its antero-posterior diameter, as well as being ong and narrow, and the respiratory movements are diminished in extent, owing to the modifications in the curvature of the ribs. The increased obliquity of the lower ribs and the falling of the shoulders also cause prominence of the scapula, giving rise to the "alar" or "pterygoid" chest of Galen and Aretaeus. Other forms of the phthinoid thorax are also described, and in many cases there are other inherited characteristics, such as delicacy of skin, fineness of hair, length of eyelashes, early development of teeth which have thin enamel and often decay early, transparency and bluish tint of conjunctivae, large pupils, rigidity of bones, with insufficient growth of their cartilages, in consequence of which they are long and slender ; precocity of intellect[1].

These outward signs are often accompanied by a certain peculiarity of constitution : weakness in resisting power, and liability to catarrhal affections and to suppuration of the lymphatic glands, on slight causes.

Heredity is also said by some writers to have a distinct influence upon the course and progress of the disease, not only in determining a certain proportion of the cases, but in hastening the period of attack[2], imparting greater severity to the disease, and in some cases increasing the tendency to haemoptysis.

There would be nothing remarkable in the fact of some hereditary predisposition to tubercle. A tendency to contract other diseases than phthisis is not infrequently transmitted from parents to children. Certain families are well known to show a peculiar susceptibility to such disorders as enteric fever and diphtheria, and most medical men have seen whole families carried off by consumption. But when we attempt to assess the exact degree to which this influence extends, we are met by several important difficulties in the way of doing this.

The members of the same family, for the most part, live under the same conditions of environment ; their house may be unhealthy, and may be favourable to the continued virulence of the bacillus of tubercle.

Boys often follow the same unhealthy occupations as their fathers ; girls live at home with their mothers, in the same possibly badly ventilated, badly drained, and ill-lighted dwellings ; and

[1] Sir W. Jenner, *Med. Times and Gazette*, 1860, I. 259 ; 1861, II. 2.
[2] Reg. Thompson, *Family Phthisis*, p. 22.

both sexes are exposed to great danger of direct infection from the habit of kissing, especially when the affected parent is the mother.

There is also increased danger of indirect infection from the tuberculous dust arising from dried-up tuberculous sputum. Under such circumstances, even persons who had no hereditary taint would be likely to contract the disease.

It is quite possible that these considerations may account for the proportions in which phthisis is supposed to have been transmitted from fathers and mothers to sons and daughters respectively; thus most observers concur in regarding the danger of transmission of the disease as greatest from father to son and from mother to daughter[1].

There is also a statistical fallacy that must be avoided in such a discussion as this. Thus the late Dr Walshe, in his Report on Pulmonary Phthisis[2], points out that, of his hospital patients, about 26 per cent. came of father or mother, or of both parents, similarly diseased ; but he does not allow that these figures prove the reality of hereditary influence, for, as he says, " This ratio of 26 per cent. might be, and probably is, no higher than that of the tuberculised portion of the population generally." " In other words, it might be predicted of any mass of individuals taken in hospitals (and of whose history nothing is known, the non-phthisical and phthisical mixed therefore) that about 26 per cent. of the generation from which they sprang were tuberculous." Hence there would be nothing in these figures to prove that their disease arose under hereditary influence.

That Dr Walshe was not far wrong may be judged from the following facts. I find, from Dr Tatham's Supplement to the Registrar-General's Fifty-fifth Report, that about two million marriages took place in the decade 1881–1890 ; the average annual death-rate per 1000, among married persons, was nearly 15 ; the total number of deaths, from twenty-five to thirty-five years of age, was about 30,000 per annum ; and the total number of deaths from phthisis, at the same ages, was 11,850 each year ;

---

[1] See table given by Dr Wilson Fox, *Diseases of the Lungs*, p. 531.
[2] *Brit. and For. Med.-Chir. Rev.* Jan. 1849.

in other words, about 39 per cent. of these deaths were from phthisis.

All these several considerations have to be taken into account in judging of the proportion of phthisical deaths that may rightly be ascribed to hereditary influence ; and, when we come to study the figures presented to us as representing this influence, we find a most bewildering discrepancy in the results.

Dr Wilson Fox[1] gives no fewer than sixteen sets of calculations of hereditary influence, but, as these vary from 4 to 66 per cent. of family influence, it does not seem to be of much use to quote them in detail.

The only safe method seems to be that employed by Dr Walshe when, as in the following table, he compared the frequency of parental taint or its absence, in the phthisical and in the non-phthisical :

	Persons themselves Phthisical	Persons non-Phthisical
Father or mother phthisical	25·94	16·55
Both father and mother free from phthisis	57·41	47·11

Dr Walshe remarks that " these results, obtained from the analysis of 446 cases, do not depose in favour of the hereditary character of the disease ; for if, on the one hand, about 9 per 100 more phthisical than non-phthisical persons came of a consumptive father or mother, on the other hand there were about 10 per 100 more phthisical than non-phthisical persons free from parental taint."

When past generations were included in the inquiry, there was slightly more evidence in favour of hereditary influence, but Dr Walshe sums up the inquiry by concluding that this influence must be very small.

It is therefore highly probable that heredity has much less to do with consumption than is popularly supposed, and that it ranks very far behind many other predisposing causes. A large proportion of cases arise without any phthisical family history in the past. Healthy families, leaving the country and coming to reside in crowded towns, often lose some members subsequently

---

[1] *Op. cit.* p. 529.

from consumption. Dr Welch has told us that, in the Army, more than 60 per cent. of the cases are non-hereditary.

We may conclude, therefore, that, with the exception of soil, none of the influences that have been now passed in review have much to do with the spread of tubercular disease, and that other causes are of much greater importance.

(3) ON CERTAIN BODILY CONDITIONS RESISTING PHTHISIS

MEDICAL CHRONICLE, *April*, 1905

HUMAN beings are classed among the animals naturally resistant to tuberculosis. Although *post-mortem* examinations show that at least 30 per cent. of mankind bear traces of the malady, this fact is really favourable to the classification, since a large proportion of the cases must have recovered without treatment, many of them without being aware of the presence of the disease.

It is probable that most healthy persons are able to resist attacks of the tubercle bacillus, if this organism is unaided by previous local injury, or by some debilitating ailment in the subject of the attack ; and the more closely the bodily condition approaches perfect health, the less likely is tubercle to take root and spread through the system. Immunity from infection is, in fact, dependent upon the efficiency of the various protective agencies of the body : the straining action of the hairs at the entrance of the air passages ; the tortuosity and the entangling mucus of these channels ; the full expansibility and elasticity of the lungs and their freedom from restraint. These safeguards prevent the lodgement of the organisms contained in tuberculous dust for sufficiently long periods to permit of pathogenic action.

In case of an actual invasion by comparatively small numbers of organisms the internal protective forces come into play, and antitoxic and phagocytic action takes place. By these means, except in the case of peculiarly susceptible persons, almost complete immunity is secured. Usually also the tubercle bacillus needs the adventitious aid of other organisms before it can penetrate the defences of the human body. But it is not only in perfect health that the human body is thus immune. It has been long recognised that there are also certain morbid conditions of the human frame which are to some extent antagonistic to tuberculosis.

The morbid conditions thus opposed to phthisis are enumerated by Dr Walshe in his work on *Diseases of the Lungs*.

R.   8

(1) Carbonaceous disease, *i.e.* anthracosis ; (2) cyanaemia ; (3) rickets ; (4) gout and calculous disease ; (5) cancer ; (6) diathetic skin disease, *e.g.* pemphigus ; (7) emphysema ; (8) nodular pulmonary apoplexy ; (9) active organic cardiac disease. Aortic aneurism. Angina. At p. 450 he says " that active cardiac disease and active tuberculosis rarely co-exist is indubitable."

Rokitansky, in his work on *Pathological Anatomy*, had already mentioned most of these pathological conditions as opposed to tubercle, and he grouped them " in a two-fold series, according as the venous habit and cyanosis are dependent upon the heart or the lungs."

He further adds (*a*) Increased density of the lungs produced by co-arctation of the thoracic spaces, *e.g.*, as in hunchbacks or some forms of spinal curvature. (This condition, however, might come under the head of rickets.) (*b*) Pleural effusion. (*c*) Pregnancy and other encroachments upon the abdominal space and the consequent narrowing of the thoracic cavity, *e.g.*, from cystic formations or dropsy ; and (*d*) Intermittent and other fevers.

Rokitansky boldly ascribes the immunity arising from all these states to the high degree of " venosity " produced by them, but he does not appear to have sufficiently verified some of his assertions.

His conclusions are several times called in question by others, notably by Dr Wilson Fox with regard to pregnancy, pleurisy, heart disease and spinal curvature. The latter author, however, expressly remarks that " conditions producing passive pulmonary congestion are adverse to the production of phthisis " ; and he illustrates his remark by reference to emphysema and heart disease. He further says : " It is a matter of common experience that, in families in whom Gout is common, phthisis is unknown[1]." He suggests that the rarity of recent tuberculosis in emphysema may be due (1) to the non-vascularity of the lungs in such cases, and atrophy of the alveolar wall ; (2) to the apical site of emphysema, and (3) to the differing age incidence of the two diseases.

Dr James Pollock, in *The Prognosis of Phthisis*, agrees that dilatation and hypertrophy of the heart, gout, and rheumatism all retard the progress of phthisis, and says that when this disease

[1] *Diseases of the Lungs*, p. 548.

is complicated with emphysema, its average is three times as long as in other cases.

Ancell, in his work *On Tuberculosis*, also discusses the partial exemption from tubercle conferred by different diseases. He dismisses cancer and, to some extent agues, but he also affirms that gout and phthisis rarely occur together. Fournet says " never." Ancell further remarks that " Tubercle is less frequently found in children who have died from rickets, than in those who have died from other diseases[1]." He considers, with Rokitansky, that chronic venosity, or defective arterialisation of the blood, however produced, seems to confer exemption from tubercular diseases.

It would perhaps be difficult to bring these allegations, as to even partial immunity, to the test of figures. Louis, James Pollock and Austin Flint are the authors who have most attempted the statistical method, and undoubtedly their results are interesting, though they can hardly be described as conclusive. So far as they go, however, they corroborate the observations of the able men already quoted : and thus we may be sure that there are strong grounds for the opinions which we have just quoted. Their conclusions are also, I think, in accord with the general experience of the profession, except perhaps Rokitansky's assertion respecting hunchbacks.

I have myself had two cases of phthisis in hunchbacks, and Dr Moritz, my colleague at the Manchester Hospital for Consumption, writes to me that he remembers two cases of hunchbacks, and remarks that: "curious to say this morning, at Hardman Street, I saw a third and fourth case with considerable kyphosis and lordosis, but not much deformity of the anterior part of the thorax," but, as he says, " after all one does not see many hunchbacks." On the whole, however, I should agree with Dr James Pollock when he remarks that deformed chest is very uncommon in phthisis and that psoriasis is rare.

I have also seen phthisis in more than one case of mitral stenosis, but whether there was compensation in these cases I cannot remember. In several instances in my own practice, pregnancy has seemed temporarily to arrest the disease, but after delivery it progressed with still greater rapidity.

[1] p. 32.

Gout and gouty skin diseases are unquestionably very rare in phthisis, and so are extreme cases of emphysema and cyanotic diseases generally, though that they do occasionally occur I can myself testify. On the whole, therefore, there are perhaps sufficient grounds for concluding that some degree of immunity from phthisis is conferred by the diseased states which have been mentioned. If so, it is natural to inquire whether there may not be some bodily condition, common to all these disorders, a condition which presents a hindrance to the entrance or the growth of the tubercle bacillus.

It seems possible that this common bodily state might be that peculiar condition which Rokitansky calls " venosity " for want of a more definite name. It means probably a plethoric condition of the capillary system of blood vessels, with imperfect reaction of the blood ; in other words, an excess of red blood-corpuscles, increased alkalinity of the blood, and increase of carbonic acid. It is difficult to say which of these conditions is chiefly antagonistic to tuberculosis, but perhaps all three are so.

In reference to the influence of alkalinity of the blood we may perhaps with advantage adduce the opinions expressed by Prof. Haliburton[1]. Speaking of the blood, he says : (1) " Venous blood contains more diffusible alkali than arterial blood, and is more bactericidal." (2) " Increase of alkalinity means increase of bactericidal power." (3) " In a condition like diabetes, where the blood is less alkaline than it should be, the susceptibility to infectious disease is increased."

" Alkalinity," he says, " is probably beneficial because it favours those oxidative processes in the cells of the body which are so essential for the maintenance of healthy life."

It is still more interesting to note that " Polycythaemia," or " cellular plethora," as it is called by Da Costa, is also common to most of the diseases which we have assumed to be hostile to the bacillus of tubercle. Thus, Da Costa notes this condition in cyanosis, peripheral stasis, as in emphysema, asphyxia, uncompensated heart disease ; and in acute paroxysm of gout, he counted over seven million corpuscles per centimetre.

In asthma also these bodies are usually in excess ; and in

---

[1] " Address on the Present Position of Physiology," *Lancet*, vol. II. 1902, p. 790.

valvular heart disease, accompanied by stasis, dyspnoea and cyanosis, a more or less decided polycythaemia is found, the count varying from six to eight millions. These changes are thought by some authors to be specially prone to occur in affections of the mitral valves. It is true that an increase of the red corpuscles takes place with inspissation of the blood from any cause, as after food, or during starvation, after diaphoresis or the action of emetics or purgatives, in diarrhoea, dysentery, etc. ; but these are usually temporary conditions which can, therefore, be easily marked off from the more permanent states of the blood.

Owing to these latter causes the count of red blood-corpuscles may also be temporarily increased in phthisis, but usually in tuberculosis, though there is a moderate loss of haemoglobin, there is little or no change in the number of red corpuscles (Da Costa).

Condition of the blood in phthisis. This point opens up another branch of the subject, namely, the state of the blood supply in phthisis in persons who are in its early stages, and in those who are progressing towards an arrest of the disease.

There is a general consensus of opinion that in the early stages of phthisis there is a diminished quantity of blood, and that the heart and aorta are small. Louis observed in 112 cases in which death was caused by phthisis, that the heart, in the majority was small, and very frequently not more than one-half or two-thirds its ordinary size. At this time also there is often some lessening in the number of the solid elements, and a deficiency of colouring matter. It is probably to this lack of haemoglobin that the grey pallor of the early consumptive is due. It is not true anaemia, and the complexion is not that of chlorosis, but is rather muddy than yellow.

The contrast to this picture presented by patients at Sanatoria towards the end of their stay is very striking. Those patients in whom the disease is arrested are for the most part florid and full of blood, approaching in many cases to actual plethora.

I have seen a number of persons who have been at Nordrach or at institutions where a similar course of forced feeding has been practised. Some of them have broken down with disordered digestions ; but most of the others had the appearance of rude health. They had not only put on flesh, but were ruddy and sunburnt, looking like farmers, some of them even more like publicans.

There could be little doubt as to their having made blood; but whether there was venous congestion or not could not well be determined. Dr Johns, however, tells me that haemorrhoids are very common amongst such patients.

It is generally understood among physicians to Sanatoria, that the course of treatment therein pursued enriches the blood both with more red corpuscles and more colouring material; but I am not aware of any definite instrumental research on these points, comparing the in-coming with the out-going patient. It is one that certainly ought to be undertaken.

I have myself made a few estimates of the red blood-corpuscles with a Gowers' Haemocyteometer, some in my own practice, and some who were kindly selected for me by Dr Johns from his Sanatorium at Alderney Manor. The results are given in the following Table, and I think the counts are fairly trustworthy, seeing that the numbers in each square varied very slightly.

Name	Age	Sex	Stage	Red Corpuscles per c.mm.	Leuco-cytes per c.mm.	Haemo-globin.	Remarks
I.	25	M	II.	4,800,000 (mean of two)	—	—	Chronic, 8 years, whole right lung diffuse T.
II.	22	M	I.	5,300,000	—	—	Early, both sides, right upper lobe, left slight.
III.	26	M	III.	5,820,000	—	—	Both lungs, right cavity and consolidation, left slight.
IV.	28	M	III.	7,600,000 (mean of two)	—	—	Left upper cavity at apex; alcoholic.
V.	22	M	I.	4,800,000	—	—	Slight physical signs. T. B. plentiful. Hæmorrhagic.
VI.	—	M	III.	6,300,000	5000	85	Cavity left apex.
VII.	26	M	II.	6,020,000	5000	81	Acute right upper lobe. Gastric troubles.
VIII.	30	F	III.	4,910,000	—	—	Two months at Stourfield Park.
IX.	40	F	III.	5,460,000	—	80	Acute right upper half cavity and consolidation.
X.	28	F	?	4,180,000	—	—	Doubtful. Rough breathing. Right apex. No T.B.
XI.	21	F	I.	4,850,000	6000	90	Slight early case. Right apex.
XII.	29	F	I.	4,675,000	7200	78	Anaemic-looking. Left apex crepitation.

Dr Coles also kindly verified my instrument by his " Thoma-Zeiss," and found it gave correct results.

It will be noticed that there are several very high readings, and that the averages of the counts are large, both for males and females. For males, the average is 5,825,000, and for females, excluding the one doubtful case, it is (4,973,750) nearly five millions. Thus, in both classes, it considerably exceeds the average in healthy persons.

It is not surprising that " erythrocytosis " should be the result of sanatorium treatment. Most of the means used certainly tend to improve the colour of the blood, and probably increase the number of red corpuscles ; such are the exposure to sunlight, the abundance of pure air and perhaps of ozone, the recumbency before and after meals. Moreover, among the circumstances enumerated by Da Costa as promoting erythrocytosis we find the use of cold baths, massage and electricity, the eating of animal food, and the resort to high altitudes[1].

In regard to the last-mentioned point, the greater resistance to tubercle which has been noted at high altitudes, and also to the well-doing of consumptives at places like Davos, St Moritz, and in the Cordillera, it is interesting to observe, as Da Costa says, " the invariable occurrence of Poly-cytosis both in the inhabitants of elevated districts and in occasional visitors, a fact still inadequately explained."

Viault estimated 8,000,000 erythrocytes in the residents on the Cordilleras, at an elevation of more than 14,000 feet above sea level. Egger estimated 7,000,000 at Arosa, at a height of 6100 feet ; and Wolff and Koeppe found an average of 5,900,000 at Reiboldsgrun at 2257 feet.

Oliver relates the interesting experience of finding in his own blood, during a stay at Davos Platz, at an elevation of 5200 feet, an increase of corpuscles within 24 hours after his arrival, the maximum estimate, 5,550,000 being attained within seven days, and the number declining within five days after his return to London.

Da Costa gives a Table, by Koeppe, illustrating the fact that

[1] Limbeck (*Syd. Soc.* vol. CLXXIV. p. 189) quotes Marestaing to the effect that sea voyages also produce an increase in the number of red corpuscles.

the higher the altitude the greater is the number of corpuscles. He himself thinks that concentration of blood explains the poly-cythaemia of high altitudes, this change being due largely to the great loss of body fluids (Grawitz), and partly to the increased arterial tension (Oliver) arising from a rarefied atmosphere.

Koeppe and others hold different views[1], but so far as our purpose is concerned the explanation is not of much importance ; the main point to be observed is that, at these high altitudes, admittedly so beneficial to consumptives, there are large propor-tions of red corpuscles in the blood.

It is not easy to account for the *preventive* influence of " venosity " of the blood, and it is still more difficult to see how it can assist the *cure* of tuberculosis.

In prevention, it may perhaps be allowable to conceive that, as Prof. Macalister shows, the venous state of the blood may cause the destruction of the bacillus on its first entrance into the body, before it has entrenched itself within a tubercle.

If a batch of tubercle bacilli, sufficiently large to cause infec-tion, should be borne into the recesses of the lungs in the form of tuberculous dust, it may lodge in an alveolus, or may even gain access into the lung tissue by way of pseudo-stomata, or by means of some local lesion, but in such a vascular organ as the lung, it will at once be brought into close relation with the blood stream, and, if the blood current is slow and the blood itself imperfectly aerated, opportunity will be given for all the bactericidal powers of both blood and tissues to be exerted upon the intruders. The disease may thus be averted at the outset.

The " cure " of the disease, when tuberculosis has been estab-lished, is a different matter. A tubercle, once formed, with its garrison of bacilli in its interior, is a kind of fortress. It is a non-vascular body. The specific organism within it is completely protected from the direct influence of the blood. The layers of exudation cells, in various stages of degeneration which surround it, are to a great extent " blood-proof," and are only penetrated by small quantities of intercellular fluids, by gases and, perhaps, by the vapours of volatile substances. All this renders it difficult to act directly upon the organism. Moreover, consumption is

[1] See also Limbeck, *loc. cit.* p. 188.

certainly not cured by deficient aeration of the blood, though, as we have seen, it is quite possible that it may be prevented thereby.

The results of " open-air " treatment show that what is needed for success is " hyper-aeration." Yet it is probable that an excess of red blood-corpuscles is as important in the cure as in the prevention of the disease. An increase in the number of these bodies, together with an increase in their contained haemoglobin, means a great power of absorption of gases, whether oxygen or CO_2.

We can thus see that " polycythaemia" may be of great importance in both cases. If oxygen, in the nascent state, is present in large quantities in the blood ; and if, owing to a plethoric stasis in the vessels, it has a longer time in which to act, arterial cellular plethora may operate in the cure of phthisis as effectually as venous plethora acts in its prevention. The mode of action in the two cases may be different, and yet they may each be assisted by an increase in the number of purveyors of gases. From these considerations then it would appear that for the " cure " of phthisis it is not " venosity " that is required, but an abundance of arterial blood, rich in all the healthy constituents of this fluid.

The quality of the blood may affect the bacillus in another way. It may, to some extent, determine the nature and quantity of the nutriment conveyed by osmose to the bacillus. If this nourishment be, as is conjectured, some volatile organic substance, such as is contained in air rendered foul by respiration, then hyperoxidation will be likely to destroy this material long before it can reach the hungry parasite.

Again, as we have seen, the condition of the blood may be able to control the admission to the tissues of other organisms, known to be the active allies of the bacillus of tubercle ; such bodies, for instance as strepto-cocci, staphylo-cocci, pneumono-cocci, and tetragonus.

If mixed infection by these and other organisms can be averted the bacillus of tubercle, in the vast majority of cases, may remain a comparatively harmless vegetable, and can be left, shut up in its own fastness, to stew in its own tuberculin until it dies. In the course of time, it will be either starved out or will lose its virulence, and the further progress of the disease will be stayed.

Phagocytosis. In considering the resisting powers of the organism, the question of phagocytosis comes naturally within our purview. In a note on this point, Dr Coles makes the following remarks :

" The introduction of a bacterial poison into the human body is attended with a reaction on the part of the white cells at the seat of injury, and in the blood system generally.

" The increase in the number of leucocytes in the blood usually bears a ratio to the degree of irritation, and by this means Nature attempts to overcome the disease.

" The process of inflammation is essentially the endeavour on the part of the organism to promote the migration of leucocytes, to aid in the inclusion and destruction of the irritant " (Sherrington).

If the irritant is small in amount or of little virulence, the reaction, as shown by the presence of leucocytosis, is also slight. When, however, the poison is overwhelming in quantity, or its virulence is great, the white cells do not increase in number, and the blood shows very little numerical alteration in its white corpuscles, and it is in these cases that a fatal determination may be expected. " In certain diseases, of which tubercle is a good example, the poison very slowly produces its effect, and no leucocytosis is generally seen. It has become a fairly universally accepted fact that ' leucocytosis does not occur in any tubercular diseases which are unattended by complications.'

" In cases of pulmonary tuberculosis, in which a pneumonic process is taking place around the original tubercular focus, or in those cases which are generally spoken of as ' mixed infections,' in which pyogenic organisms are present, the leucocytes in the blood are frequently greatly increased in number."

It is probable that the white blood-corpuscle, as seen in blood or tissues, has the power of attacking living bacteria, and by that means rendering them harmless. More recent observers, especially Hankin and Kanthack, have shown that the white corpuscles also produce their beneficial effect by secreting substances (" Alexines ") which are toxic to the germs.

Now, at this point comes in the influence of sanatorium treatment, and especially its influence upon the blood. In order to increase the fighting power of the leucocytes of the body, it is essential to render the body generally, and the leucocytes in particular, as fit as possible. This is attained by the modern treatment of phthisis by pure air, good feeding, rest, etc.

In a valuable paper by Dr Galbraith[1], he says : " In cases treated by the open-air method and on a diet rich in animal nitrogen, the characteristic features of the blood-counts are (1) a moderate, constant leucocytosis, (2) a large absorptive lymphocytosis, and (3) an almost constant eosinophilia ; the eosinophile cells varying from 4 per cent. to 5 per cent. of the total leucocytes. The total number of the leucocytes varied, in one case, from 10,000 at 8 a.m. to 19,000 at 3 p.m. This exceptionally large increase occurred after two meals consisting mainly of nitrogenous food."

He further remarks : " If it be true that the leucocytes have a special anti-bacterial action, and that changes in them are evidence of a reaction to poisoning, which may be common to all tissues, but is demonstrable only in the blood, then only those constituents of the diet which are known to produce or favour this reaction need be in excess of the normal." Again, " a diet mainly animal furnishes the largest amount of nuclein derivatives in proportion to the quantity taken, while, if properly administered, it throws least strain upon the organism."

Dr Coles remarks further : " Some investigators have considered that the leucocytes in the blood of phthisical patients should be stimulated. To some extent the so-called ' sun-baths ' accomplish this."

As Buchner says : " The injection of various substances, such as physiological saline solution, bouillon, etc., into the body of a guinea pig may be followed by a temporary increase of the natural resistance which may even simulate a specific immunisation."

Landerer has for several years successfully treated phthisis by the injection of cinnamic acid, an agent that produces leucocytosis.

Others have given, for the same purpose, yeast, nuclein, or similar substances by the mouth, and have claimed to have

---

[1] *Brit. Med. Journ.* March 14th, 1903, p. 600.

obtained very decided improvements by these means. Perhaps also the use of blisters comes within the same category.

In any case, it may be safely said that such methods are based on a scientific principle, next only in importance to the attempt, so far unsuccessful, of rendering the bacillus of tubercle, *in situ*, inert.

The composition and the extent of the bactericidal power of the blood may thus become of extreme importance in the cure of consumption.

I believe that the success of sanatorium treatment may indeed to some extent be explained by its blood-making power, a power which may even have to be pushed beyond the limits of perfect health. I am aware that this is not the explanation usually given. The popular theory is that, by purely hygienic means, the health of the patient is so completely restored that his tissues and his blood are able to make a successful stand against the attacks of the bacillus.

Doubtless the restoration to the consumptive of such a degree of health as is possible to him must improve his power of resistance to the microbe; but I consider that sanatorium treatment does far more than merely improve the general health, and thus that it deserves something more significant than the title of " Traitement Hygiénique," given to it by some French authors.

Each factor of the sanatorium treatment has indeed a distinctly remedial as well as a hygienic aim. Thus :

1. The abundance of fresh air and sunshine, and the measures of disinfection practised in all sanatoria, create an almost " aseptic atmosphere," and banish most pathogenic organisms from the immediate environment of the patient.

2. The prolonged periods of absolute recumbent rest prescribed for all acute cases give the greatest possible measure of immobility to the ribs over the inflamed portions of the lungs. This rest, together with the absence of irritation by dust or organic matter in the air, soothes cough and reduces fever.

3. The graduated exercises and massage improve appetite, and thus tend to increase weight, and assist the other measures in improving the general tone, in other words the nerve power of the subject.

4. The large allowance of food of all kinds and especially of
fats and strong animal food, causes, in most cases, a great increase
in weight; thus also increasing the hopefulness and buoyancy
of spirit in the patient.

It may be affirmed, therefore, that each of the factors in
sanatorium treatment takes part, not only in the hygienic improvement of the patient's condition, but also in a direct attack upon
the disease itself.

May there not, however, be something more in this treatment
than has hitherto been recognised. It is remarkable, to say the
least, how all the before-mentioned agents in the cure combine,
as if in a sort of converging fire, to bring about that very condition of "cellular plethora" which we have seen to constitute
so potent a protection against tubercle. Fresh air and sunshine,
rest in bed, a full animal diet, baths and massage, elevation above
the sea (and sea voyages), all these, as we have seen, promote a
state of "Polycythaemia."   We may then inquire (1) is the
success obtained in some sanatoria in any way due to the induction
of this condition ? and (2) is it a point that may legitimately be
aimed at ?

These are important questions which cannot well be answered
without much more research, but I venture to submit that they
are worthy of consideration, and that it would be well if the
managers of sanatoria would permit the necessary investigation.

SECTION III. RESEARCHES

(1) THE INFLUENCE OF IODOFORM ON THE BODY-WEIGHT IN PHTHISIS[1]

British Medical Journal, *January* 3, 1884.

ABOUT a year ago, iodoform was introduced to the English medical public, mainly by Dr Dreschfeld, as a drug likely to be of service in the treatment of phthisis, when used internally and by means of inhalation. I determined last year to give it a trial at the Hospital for Consumption in Manchester. At first, I met with some disappointment; many persons, especially women, were unable to take it in consequence of the nausea and disturbance of the digestive organs that it caused. However, I still persevered, and gave it in the form of a pill, a grain and a half three times a day, to all the cases of phthisis who could take it. Shortly afterwards, at the suggestion of Dr Marsh, I combined it with two grains of croton-chloral, and found that it was then much better borne by the patients, both male and female. Iodine and iodoform inhalations were also prescribed as a general test of its influence upon the disease. The weight of the patients was recorded for some little time before its use, and after its administration; and on the accompanying charts I have traced curves showing the loss or gain in weight during the treatment.

It seemed better to make no selection of cases; and it was given at all stages of the disease; and as patients seldom presented themselves in the incipient stage, the largest number of cases were in the more advanced stages of phthisis. The drug in several cases was stopped for various causes, and again recommenced.

Owing to the causes that I have mentioned, there are only 21 complete cases recorded at the present time. Of these, 4 were in the first, 5 in the second, and 12 in the third stage of the disease.

---

[1] This paper was accompanied by charts showing the progress of each case under the use of iodoform.

Of the 4 cases in the first stage, 3 appear to have received
benefit ; one (R. Jones) gained 2½ lbs. in three weeks, and maintained her position for at least six weeks afterwards ; another
(S. Menzies) gained 2 lbs. in about one month, and although she
lost weight somewhat on discontinuing the drug, she regained it
again when the pills were recommenced. A third case (E. Lancell)
gained 11 lbs. in four months, and was then lost sight of. The
fourth (M. Clevorty) lost weight on the whole to the extent of
8 lbs. in three months.

Of the 5 cases in the second stage of the disease, No. 1 (McMillen)
was losing weight rapidly, when he commenced the treatment, at
the rate of 3 lbs. in a fortnight ; he then gained 1 lb. in the same
space of time ; lost weight on discontinuing the drug, gained
again slightly on its recommencement, lost ground a third time
on its omission, and entered on the third stage in about three
months from the beginning of the treatment ; but after again
taking iodoform for several weeks, he improved and regained his
former weight.

No. 2 (Ross) also took the drug intermittingly ; he gained
2½ lbs. in ten days after first taking it ; but after this it seemed
to have little influence in arresting his downward course.

No. 3 (Brackenridge) presented a similar history, except that,
in spite of sundry alternations of weight, he had on the whole
gained somewhat in the course of seven months' treatment,
during which time he had only omitted the iodoform for about
three weeks.

No. 4 (Lockett) was a case of chronic pneumonia, which
developed into phthisis after a lapse of four months. He was
losing weight rapidly when he commenced the iodoform-pills ;
but since then he has gradually improved both in weight and in
the condition of the lungs.

No. 5 (Matthews) has only been a short time under treatment ;
but he has gained 3½ lbs. in the first fortnight.

Of the 12 cases in the third stage of the complaint, 2 (Burns
and Burke) have distinctly gained weight since taking iodoform.
Six, after sundry variations, remain approximately at the same
weight, several after six or eight months of the treatment. The
remaining 4 have all diminished in weight, with more or less

rapidity. It is, however, remarkable that, even in these advanced cases, there is often a temporary rise for a short time after commencing to take the iodoform. Thus I note that, after a total number of 35 times of such administration, there were 28 periods in which there was an increase of weight, and only 7 in which the loss of weight continued without intermission.

From a review of all the cases, I am inclined, therefore, to attribute to iodoform some slight improvement, even in cases in which it was manifestly hopeless to expect cure ; and I think that, in the earlier stages of the disease, it is decidedly worthy of further trial.

January 2nd, 1884. Since the above observations were made (August 1883), the same treatment has been pursued in many other cases presenting themselves at the hospital, with very similar results.

2) ON INTRAPULMONARY INJECTIONS

MEDICAL CHRONICLE, *January*, 1887

A PAPER was read at the Annual Meeting of the British Medical Association, at Cardiff, in 1885, by Dr Shingleton Smith, upon the Intrapulmonary Injection of Iodoform (published in *Brit. Med. Journal* for 1885, Vol. II. p. 813). A few of the cases admitted into the Hospital for Consumption seemed to be well suited for a trial of this treatment, and a record of the results may be found interesting to those who have read the previous paper. The following notes are abridged from those taken by Dr Milne, the resident medical officer.

1. *Gangrene of the Lung.*—Mrs W., æt. 33, married, six children, admitted October 1st, 1885. There is no family history of consumption. Had pleuro-pneumonia when 14 months old, and since then has always suffered from winter cough. After each of her last four confinements had an attack of acute pleurisy. Her last child was born 19 months ago, and the attack then lasted two months. About six months before admission she had an attack of acute pneumonia, which left a permanent consolidation of the base of the right lung posteriorly. About three weeks after admission into the hospital, during which time she lost 4½ lbs. in weight, she had a sharp feverish attack ; the breath was offensive, and the sputum, which had been frothy and muco-purulent, became excessively fœtid, and of a dark prune juice colour. There was some dyspnœa, and pain on both sides of the chest posteriorly. Temperature, 101° F. On examination there was found slight dulness on percussion in both the supra-spinous regions, and at the right base posteriorly, from the eighth to the twelfth rib, complete absence of resonance, and on the left side, in one spot, there was hyper-resonance. On auscultation there was heard cavernous breathing, gurgling râles and pectoriloquy over the dull area on the right side, especially in the middle of this region, and on the left side there was bronchial breathing and some bronchophony, with mucous râles, except over an area about two inches in diameter, near the level of the tenth rib, in

R.   9

the scapular line, and here the breathing was cavernous with bubbling râles. The breath sounds at both apices were slightly impaired. The chest measurements were 14½ inches on the left, and 15¾ inches on the right, in a line just above the nipples. The expansion was equal on the two sides. Heart normal. Naturally there was much suspicion of tubercle, but after repeated examinations, no bacilli were found in the sputum, but in one specimen there were seen numerous micrococci, both in masses and in chains. It was concluded, therefore, that the case was one of gangrene of the right base, and, after some hesitation, it was assumed that the cavity on the left side was due to bronchiectasis. She was ordered iron and quinine, and inhalations of carbolic acid from hot water, and eucalyptus oil on respirator inhaler. These means somewhat diminished the fœtor of the breath and of the sputum, and two days later 10 minims of an ethereal solution of iodoform (1 gr. in 5 minims) were injected into the cavity on the right side. A similar injection was made daily into this cavity, except upon two days when it was injected into the left cavity, where it caused much more pain than on the right. After two days of this treatment it was noted that the sputum had lost its prune juice colour, and was less offensive. The patient felt better, but the cough and the amount of muco-purulent expectoration remained excessive. On November 14th a dose of 10 minims of ol. eucalypti was ordered thrice daily, and on the 16th it was noted that the expectoration was more frothy in character, but on the 18th it again became prune juice coloured and offensive. On November 24th further improvement was noted, and on Nov. 28th the injections were discontinued until December 2nd, when in place of the ethereal solution, an emulsion of iodoform in olive oil was used, with much less pain to the patient, and this treatment was continued, with intervals of a few days, for several weeks, during which time she gained about 10 lbs. in weight, and improved greatly in her general health, though the signs of a cavity in each lung still continued. Upon one occasion the injection needle used was rather a large one, and apparently it pierced some large vein, for a little blood exuded when the needle was withdrawn, and there was copious hæmoptysis for a few minutes. After her recovery from this accident she went out of the hospital for a fortnight, and after a short stay as an in-patient, in April, she went to Southport for a month. At the present time (October, 1886) the bronchiectasis has disappeared, and though the cavity in the right lung is still perceptible, she has no cough nor expectoration, and appears to be in good health. The other cases in which the intra-pulmonary treatment was tried were all of them phthisical.

2. R. R., æt. 18, was a patient of Dr Simpson's, who kindly allows me to mention his case. This boy had a vomica at the apex of the left lung, near the surface, and iodoform in ether was twice injected into it, but as it caused much pain and distress, without any apparent benefit, the treatment was discontinued.

3. H. W., æt. 35, butcher, admitted November 26th, 1885. Phthisis not hereditary. The previous history of undoubted lung disease was only four months, and in that time he had lost 28 lbs. in weight, but he had only coughed for one month. His sputum was loaded with bacilli, but as the case was so recent, and as he had a vomica at the apex of the left lung, very near the surface, it was thought that it might prove to be a case favourable for injection. For a fortnight, therefore, 15 minims of a solution of iodoform in oil of eucalyptus was injected every second or third day. No bad effects followed, and he expressed himself as some-what relieved by the treatment, and gained 4 lbs. in weight in the first week ; but after this it became evident that general tuber-culosis had set in, and the injections were discontinued. He remained in hospital until January 8th, and then went home, and his death was reported to us about a month afterwards.

4. W. P., æt. 18, a railway advertising agent, admitted March 18th, 1886. No family history of phthisis. Had coughed for about four months, and during the last month has had slight hæmoptysis at intervals. The signs of tubercular disease were confined to about three inches of the right apex, where there was also a small vomica near the surface, just under the clavicle. This vomica was injected four times, at intervals of two days, with 10 minims of a solution of iodoform in oil of eucalyptus (1 in 6). On the last occasion, after about 4 minims had been injected, he said he felt it " going all through him." His face became pale, his pupils dilated, his breathing hurried, pulse quick.

He complained of an aching in his limbs, especially the legs, and of a pricking sensation in his fingers. He said he felt " as if about to die." His cheeks soon became flushed, and there were several irregular patches of erythema on the trunk and limbs. Within five minutes of the injection there appeared several well-marked patches of urticaria on the chest and back. In another five minutes these, along with the spots of erythema, had all disappeared ; his pulse and breathing now became slower, and he soon felt all right again, with the exception of slight aching in the head and legs. About twelve hours afterwards he had an epileptic fit of some severity, and remained dazed and slightly incoherent for some time. He had two slighter fits at five hours' intervals afterwards, and between the seizures he complained of frontal headache, but otherwise felt quite well. We could not ascertain that the injections had in any way affected the course of the disease.

5. Mary H., æt. 16, house servant, admitted March 6th, 1886. History of phthisis on the father's side. Has had cough for six months, and has been getting thinner and shorter of breath during this period. Consolidation of the left apex to the fifth rib continuously was noted, and a small vomica under the clavicle ; no other signs of lung disease.

On April 10th, the vomica was injected with ten minims of a solution of iodoform in oil of eucalyptus, and on April 20th the injection was repeated. These injections produced a good deal of pain at the site of the puncture, lasting about twelve hours.

On April 22nd, in the early morning, the patient awoke with a severe fit of coughing, when she suddenly felt a sharp pain over the site of the vomica, and this was followed by signs of pneumo-thorax on the left side, but three weeks later it is noted that these signs had entirely disappeared, though the vomica remained the same size as previously.

She stayed in the hospital six weeks longer, and gained 5 lbs. in weight, and seemed much better in general health, but this improvement can hardly be ascribed to the iodoform injections.

I have since ascertained that the disease is making slow progress.

Remarks.—The injections of iodoform were made, for the most part, with one of Mayer and Meltzer's syringes, having a strong gilt needle. This was inserted between the ribs, near the upper margin of the lower one ; care was then taken to ascertain if the end of the needle had reached the cavity, or at any rate an air space, by withdrawing the piston, and unless air bubbled through the fluid, the needle was moved slightly until this sign of its having penetrated into an air channel was perceived. The njection was then completed.

In the case of gangrene of the lung, it was necessary to pierce the intercostal space in the dorsal region, where the ribs were rather close together, and this fact, together with the large size of the needle, may have had something to do with the occurrence of hæmorrhage, though my impression is that the instrument traversed some very congested vessels near the seat of the disease, and not that an intercostal vessel had been wounded.

In Case 4, in spite of the precautions taken, the drug must have been injected into the circulatory system, and the alarming nature of the symptoms produced shows the necessity for great caution in the operation.

In Case 5, in which pneumo-thorax occurred two days after the puncture, it is possible that the wound may have opened slightly and that some air may have escaped into the pleura by this track, but on the other hand, it may have taken place in the ordinary course of the disease. Even if it was due to the operation however, this accident need not deter us from its performance. The simple pneumo-thorax so produced would probably do more good than harm, and would give temporary rest to the diseased lung.

It will have been observed that the only case in which the treatment was thoroughly carried out was the case of gangrene, and this patient was the only one in which we could ascribe direct benefit to the iodoform injection. There can be little doubt, I think, that the favourable course of the disease in this case was mainly due to the treatment by injection and in a similar case I should certainly repeat the experiment.

In Dr R. Shingleton Smith's case of gangrene, although temporary improvement followed the injections of iodoform, the case terminated fatally ; and in the case of chronic pneumonia the treatment was also unsuccessful.

In the tubercular cases, the number of injections in each varied from two to eight, and it is probable that some good effect was temporarily produced in Cases 3 and 5, but on the whole the results were not encouraging. I observe that of Dr Smith's three cases of this disease, only one, into which nine injections were made, showed any marked improvement from the treatment. It is probable that to effectually disinfect a tuberculous lung many more injections would have to be made than we have attempted so far, and it is doubtful whether many patients would be found to submit to it. Apart from the danger of accidents such as have been mentioned, the procedure is somewhat alarming and dis-agreeable to the patients. The ethereal solution was very painful, and the olive oil emulsion was so viscid that a larger needle had to be employed than was absolutely safe. The solution of iodo-form in oil of eucalyptus was quite the most satisfactory of all the mixtures that were tried.

(3) NOTES ON THE TREATMENT OF PHTHISIS BY PURE OXYGEN AND OZONISED OXYGEN

Read before the Manchester Medical Society, February 15, 1888

MONSIEUR PASTEUR has shown the power of the oxygen and ozone of the atmosphere in attenuating the infective power of various micro-organisms. The good effects also of fresh air, both in the treatment of consumption and in its prevention, have now been placed beyond a doubt.

It was on these grounds thought desirable that a thorough trial should be given to oxygen and ozone at the Manchester Hospital for Consumption and Diseases of the Throat.

It may be said that something had already been done towards this end in the construction and aeration of the wards of the hospital at Bowdon. In the older portion of the building, 6000 cubic feet of fresh warmed air are admitted per head per hour, and in addition to this large supply the windows of both wards and living rooms are kept open winter and summer, night and day. There are also several Tobin's ventilators in each room.

In the two new pavilion wards, erected by Mr W. F. Crossley, still larger amounts of fresh warmed air are constantly passed through the ventilator, and, if required, 18,000 cubic feet of air can be admitted per head per hour. It has been ascertained also that the entering air contains a fair amount of ozone.

The results of this large admission of pure air from the gardens of the institution upon the health of the patients have, on the whole, been very satisfactory. In most of the cases admitted, there has been at least a temporary arrest of the activity of the disease, attested by the diminution of fever, by a gain in weight, and by the absence of night sweats. Owing to the kindness of Messrs Dewhurst an opportunity has, however, been afforded of trying the effects of Brin's pure oxygen in the treatment of certain selected cases. Since February, 1887, no less than twenty-four cylinders, each containing twenty cubic feet of pure oxygen, have been supplied to the institution without charge.

Moreover, two dozen syphons of oxygenated water and some bottles of milk were provided for the use of patients.

The inhalations were not given directly from the cylinders, but a Claver's nitrous oxide inhaler was used. After the bag had been filled with oxygen, the current was shut off, and the patient allowed to exhaust the contained quantity, expiration being performed into the external air through an aperture with a valve opening outwards.

The following notes as to the action of pure oxygen were made by Mr Cottam, Resident Medical Officer at the Institution :

Inhalation.—Three patients inhaled pure oxygen for periods of time beginning with five minutes, and gradually increasing up to fifteen.

(1) K. W., a case of phthisis ; third stage, on left chest, early second on the right ; bacilli had been found in the sputum. She inhaled oxygen almost every day for four weeks in the manner stated above. The pulse and respiration were both diminished in number at the end of the experiment. These effects were very temporary, and were very possibly exaggerated by nervousness. The patient said she felt clearer and lighter after an inhalation ; and on two occasions a headache was cleared away. If given just before a meal, the appetite was improved. No effect, as far as could be ascertained, upon the bacilli.

(2) S. H. In this case the left apex was breaking down ; the right showed slight consolidation in the same region. There was a marked family history of phthisis.

The result of a week's inhalations was almost inappreciable. Pulse and respiration unaffected. Appetite slightly improved and there was the same feeling of clearness as in the case of K. W. Patient was usually sleepy after an inhalation.

(3) M. H. This patient's lungs were both in the third stage of phthisis, the left being more advanced. Bacilli were found in the sputum.

On inhalation, pulse and respiration were both increased at first, afterwards diminished. The patient was liable to headaches, and these always disappeared after respiring oxygen, and she felt lighter and brighter. The respiratory power distinctly increased after a short period of inhalation. No effect could be observed upon the number of bacilli.

In these three well-marked cases of phthisis the inhalations were never found to excite coughing unless the patient took a very deep inspiration ; but a deep inspiration in ordinary air produced just as much coughing.

Oxygenated Water.—This was given alone or with milk. In cases where there was gastric irritability, with pain or discomfort after food, or where there was vomiting independently of coughing, milk and oxygenated water were easily retained, and almost invariably without discomfort, and there was no objection on the part of the patients to taking oxygenated water. Depressant after-effects were never noticed.

Oxygenated Milk.—This did not get a fair trial, for it was found impossible to keep it for more than a few days after arrival.

Ozone.—Whilst these observations upon the action of pure oxygen were being carried out, it was also thought desirable to ascertain the effect of ozonising the pure gas as it issued from the cylinders. It was thought possible that the deleterious effects of ozone, that had been at various times observed by others, might have been due partly to some impurity. Ozone was accordingly obtained by connecting the wires from an induction coil with the inner and outer tubes of an ozone-generator (Tinsley's), and allowing a gentle stream of oxygen from a Brin's cylinder to pass through the tubes. The apparatus was at first placed in the ventilating chamber, underneath one of the pavilion wards. By means of test papers ozone could be found passing into the ward in increased quantity, but as no appreciable results followed, and, as, moreover, atmospheric ozone was found in considerable quantities in the air entering the ventilating chamber by its louvres, this method was soon discontinued. It was then tried in the sunbath with nine, ten, or a dozen patients, with the windows closed, for half an hour. Irregular results were obtained from pulses and respirations, and there was marked increase in coughing and headaches (? probably due in part to confinement of excess of patients in a limited area).

Similar treatment in a small ward with three or four patients at the most, and continuing for about six weeks, gave the following results : The room used was 2790 cubic feet in size. The patients were left in the room for an hour, with the exception of J. S., who remained usually half an hour. The general effects observed were these : Sleepiness (only one patient out of five unaffected) ; increased appetite for the next meal ; no marked effect on either pulse or respiration ; no irritable effects, such as increased coughing ; no headache ; no definite alteration in the amount of bacilli in sputa. One patient (G. H.) was brought in for one inhalation, but coughed so much that it was not thought advisable to continue in his case. L. C. felt very little difference during several weeks trial, though she could readily detect by the smell the presence of ozone. On two occasions the stream of pure oxygen was shut off, and the ozone obtained from ordinary air. On both occasions *all* the patients complained of coughing and a sense of irritation.

Pure Ozone under slight pressure.—Mr Cottam and I then tried the effect of inhaling pure ozonised oxygen that had been passed into a Waldenberg's apparatus—a kind of gasometer upon which more or less pressure could be made by means of weights and counter weights. As we experienced no ill effects from our inhalation, I selected the following case as one upon whom cautiously graduated experiments with this gas could be tried. The notes have been furnished to me by Mr Cottam.

A. J. E., aged 49, of good family history, was admitted Oct. 10th, 1887. His previous history was as follows : Winter cough since 1882, usually quite well in the summer. Last spring the cough, instead of leaving him, increased. His breathing became shorter, and he lost flesh. The expectoration became freer, and changed from a frothy black and white to a yellowish green. No hæmoptysis and no night sweats. On admission it was found that the apex of the left lung was beginning to break down, but no definite signs of a cavity could be detected. Moist râles could be heard down to the base of the fifth dorsal spine behind. Bacilli in moderate numbers were found in the sputum, which was thick and muco-purulent. After he had been in hospital seven weeks, during which time he gained some 7 lbs. in weight, he was given inhalations of oxygen and ozone under pressure. A stream of oxygen, driven through an ozoniser, had about 8 per cent. of its volume converted into ozone by means of a current from an induction coil and battery. The mixture of oxygen and ozone was passed into the pneumatic apparatus, holding (during this series of experiments) 560 cubic inches.

December 5th.—The patient was given two inhalations under a pressure of 3 kilos (6½ lbs.) at first, and the amount was gradually increased to four inhalations at 4 kilos (9 lbs.) pressure, daily, during a period of five weeks. The following observations were made. There was no difference between the pulse taken before inhalation and that taken after, and none in the number of respirations. The patient felt brighter and more buoyant, and after a few days could walk further and with more comfort, slept better, appetite markedly improved, especially for breakfast and tea. Increase in weight between 5 and 6 lbs. (he was taking cod liver oil during the whole period). Increased respiratory power, gauged by lessening the number of respirations in which he was able to empty the ozone chamber. No catarrh ; and at no time could any irritating effects be noticed. He never coughed, either at the beginning or at the end of inhalation. The ordinary morning cough and expectoration diminished. At the end of the first week bacilli could not be found in the sputum, and when again examined at intervals four times subsequently, bacilli were absent. Two other patients (males) were also submitted to daily ozonised inhalations, but it will be unnecessary to give the details of their cases. One—B. H., æt. 29—had been admitted as an in-patient three months before this special treatment was commenced. He had a small cavity in the left apex, and infiltration to four inches below the clavicle, and on the right side, under the upper three ribs, and under the supra-spinous fossa behind, the lung was undergoing softening. He had already improved very much in health during his stay in the Hospital, having gained nearly 13 lbs. in weight, and he had no fever or night sweats, but the bacilli in the sputum were numerous. He has now had daily inhalations for three weeks, emptying Waldenberg's gaso-meter at first twice, and then three times at each sitting, the contents being 633 cubic inches each time. He continued to gain in weight, and expresses himself as feeling much better since the treatment was commenced. Sleeps, eats, and breathes much better ; the temperature is normal, and the pulse has diminished in rate from 80 to 70. The sputum has been twice examined, on January 29th and February 12th, and on each occasion many bacilli still appeared.

J. T. J., æt. 19, had phthisis in the second stage on the right, and probably slight consolidation on the left side. He commenced the inhalations on January 20th, having been in hospital ten days. His weight on January 20th was 110½ lbs., and on February 15th it was 115 lbs. He emptied the cylinder under a pressure of 4 kilos, from two to five times, and seems to have benefited from the treatment. His pulse also has slowed somewhat ; he eats and sleeps better, and his temperature is normal. His sputum, examined on January 30th, showed no bacilli, but on February 14th a few were found.

I have ventured to publish these few imperfect notes, not because I think they afford any conclusive proof of the action of oxygen or of ozone upon tubercle, for this proof can only be obtained by a much longer study of the subject, but because I think that certain of the facts already ascertained are worthy of notice, and because by their statement, other observers may be induced to repeat and to carry further these observations, as I certainly mean to do myself. It has thus been ascertained (1) that pure oxygen, without any admixture of air, may be inhaled continuously for at least 15 minutes, and probably for a longer period, without the slightest harm resulting, without producing inflammation, or even irritation of the air passages, without increase of fever, or even elevation of the pulse-rate. (2) It has been proved that from 2000 to 4000 cubic inches of pure ozonised oxygen may be breathed, not only without harm, but even with apparent benefit in the cases in which it was tried. (3) If we may trust our repeated microscopic examinations, the ozone diminished the number of bacilli in the expectoration in two cases, and in the third, the expectoration was diminished. and the disease was quiescent. The general condition of the patients was much improved.

March 19th.—The patient, A. J. E., went out of hospital on January 30th. He came for several weeks to the Dispensary, and seemed still to be improving, and he was gaining weight ;

but on March 5th I was informed that he had died suddenly of hæmoptysis.

Patients B. H. and J. T. J. are still under treatment, and are gaining weight steadily. In each case the disease seems to be stationary, but microscopical examination still shows bacilli in the sputum.

(4) ON CERTAIN CONDITIONS THAT MODIFY THE VIRULENCE OF THE BACILLUS OF TUBERCLE

PROCEEDINGS OF THE ROYAL SOCIETY, VOL. XLIX.

Read November 29, 1890

IT is acknowledged by most pathologists that tubercular sputum, dried up and broken into dust, is the most common vehicle by which the bacillus of tubercle is conveyed into the body.

But its power for evil is obviously modified by a multitude of conditions, some of them inherent in the animal body exposed to infection, others due to external influences. Judging from the facts relating to the distribution of tubercular disease, its incidence in certain localities, and especially its prevalence in badly drained, badly ventilated, and imperfectly lighted dwellings, it has been surmised that the three chief external conditions that mitigate the virulence of the bacillus are : (1) a dry soil, (2) abundance of fresh air, and (3) light.

But hitherto, few, if any, direct experiments have been made to determine the extent to which these several influences possess mitigating powers.

It is true that Dr Candler, in his work on the Prevention of Consumption, affirms that light is the chief agent in destroying the bacillary virus, and Professor Koch, in his address to the International Congress at Berlin this year, lends the weight of his great authority to the same opinion ; but, in neither case, is any proof given of the truth of this view[1].

It was in order to test the influence of light, air, and dry soils upon the virulence of the bacillus of tubercle that the following series of experiments was devised.

[1] [Since this was written, I have learnt that Savitzly has ascertained that phthisical sputum, exposed "at the ordinary room temperature, and generally under all common life conditions," retains its infectiousness not longer than 2½ months, and, other conditions being equal, a sputum dried in darkness loses its infectious properties within the same period as a sputum exposed to light. *Med. Chronicle,* Nov. 1890, p. 117.]

It was decided to expose tuberculous sputum :

(*a*) In a locality (Bowdon) where the soil was dry and sandy (about 100 feet in thickness) and where very few cases of phthisis were known to have originated. It was to be placed in full daylight or sunlight, and exposed to abundant streams of fresh country air.

(*b*) A portion of the same sputum would be exposed under similar conditions, in the same place, with the exception that it would be put into a darkened chamber.

(*c*) A third portion would be taken to a small four-roomed tenement in Manchester, on a clay soil, without cellarage—and badly ventilated, but it would be placed on the window ledge, with as much light as could there be obtained.

(*d*) A portion would be placed in the same cottage, but in a dark corner of a sleeping room in which it was known that three deaths from phthisis had occurred within the space of six or seven years.

(*e*) Finally, a portion would be exposed to used air coming from a ward in a Consumption Hospital, in Bowdon, in darkness. These intentions were fully carried out.

Two collections of sputum were obtained :

A. From a woman dying of phthisis, collected on April 25. This specimen contained comparatively few bacilli.

B. Also from a woman in an advanced stage of phthisis, collected on April 27. This sputum contained abundance of bacilli.

Sputum (A) was not considered to be very suitable for the purpose owing to the sparseness of bacilli ; but it was decided to use it by way of control experiment ; owing to an accident, the portions exposed under conditions (*c*) and (*d*) were lost.

These collections of sputum were divided into portions, and placed in watch glasses marked A 1, A 2, A 3, B 1,......, B 10. Some of these watch glasses were exposed without further arrangement, but others, where there might be a possibility of infection, were enclosed in cages, so arranged that air could reach them through a thin layer of cotton wool, one kind of cage being constructed of two squares of glass, supported at their edges by cork, and surrounded by cotton wool, the other of small flasks the bottom of which had been cut off, and the lower edge resting in a small circular tray fitted with wool, the mouths of the flasks being also loosely stuffed with the wool.

These watch glasses were then exposed for five weeks under the conditions already noted, commencing on April 29, 1890, with the exception of B 9 and 10, which were started on May 2. Most of the specimens were withdrawn on June 3 ; but one, B 10, was divided on May 13, and a portion, B 10*a*, was introduced into a glass bulb and exposed for several minutes each day to a current of ozonised oxygen.

All the specimens were then enclosed in a box and forwarded to the Pathological Laboratory, Owens College, where Dr Dreschfeld, the Professor of Pathology, had kindly undertaken to carry out the necessary inoculations. Owing to various causes, some of these operations were not commenced until June 27, 1890, others not until July 10. The animals used were rabbits, kept under favourable hygienic conditions. The dried sputum was mixed with sterilised water, to form a pasty mass, and this was inserted into the subcutaneous tissue of the back. All the instruments used were made thoroughly aseptic.

The following tables give :
    (1)   The conditions of exposure.
    (2)   The date of inoculation.
    (3)   The date of death, by killing or otherwise.
    (4)   Dr Dreschfeld's report upon the results of the inoculation.

TABLE I.—*Influence of Dry Soil, Air, and Light*

No. of specimen.	Conditions of exposure.	Date of Inoculation.	Death.	Dr Dreschfeld's reports.
A 1	In outdoor studio, Bowdon. In light and free ventilation in flask arrangement	June 27	Killed Sept. 4	Rabbit in good condition; wound completely healed cicatrix of wound scarcely visible. All inserted sputum completely disappeared, only a few pigmented streaks left, no caseation; internal organs healthy.
A 2	Ditto, open watchglass	July 10	Killed Sept. 4	In good condition; wound healed, good cicatrix no caseous mass. In liver a number of disseminated firm spots; microscopically, these consisted of fibrous tissue; no tubercle bacilli found in them.
B 6	Ditto in cotton wool cage	July 10	Killed Sept. 4	In good condition; cicatrix healed, no trace of sputum left, no caseation where sputum had been inoculated, only a few pigmented streaks.
B 7	Ditto in open cage until May 9, then cotton wool added	July 10	Killed Sept. 4	Good condition; cicatrix perfect, some fibrous induration in subcutaneous tissue where sputum had been; no caseation; internal organs healthy.

TABLE II.—*Influence of Dry Soil, Air, and Darkness*

No. of speci-men.	Conditions of exposure.	Date of Inocu-lation.	Date of Death.	Dr Dreschfeld's reports.
A 3	In darkened photo-graphic room, Bow-don, in watch-glass	June 27	Killed Sept. 4	Rabbit; in good condition, small caseous mass be-neath healed wound; all internal organs healthy. Microscopic examination of caseous mass.—Granu-lar detritus, no tubercle bacilli.
B 8	Ditto in cotton wool cage	June 27	Died Aug. 26	Moderately emaciated; wound healed, but the edges separated on pulling the skin at the sides. In the subcutaneous tissue beneath the wound a few yellowish, soft spots, about the size of pin-heads, surrounded by a zone of hyperæmia. Inter-nally all organs healthy, no signs of tubercle, right heart full of blood, left heart empty. Microscopic examination of the yel-low spots shows them to consist of granular detri-tus and a few granule cells; no tubercle bacilli could be detected.
B 9	Under ward of Con-sumptive Hospital in full ventilation, in darkness, in cotton wool cage	July 10	Died Aug. 14	Emaciated; wound healed under a scab, a thin mass of yellow caseous mate-rial just beneath the skin. Heart and lungs healthy; kidneys contained a num-ber of small cysts. In the caseous mass *a few tu-bercle bacilli were found.*

TABLE III.—*Influence of Clay Soil, Bad Air, and Light*

No. of specimen.	Conditions of exposure.	Date of Inoculation.	Death.	Dr Dreschfeld's reports.
B 3	On window-sill of small cottage bedroom in Ancoats. Flask arrangement	June 27	Died Aug 14	Large rabbit; emaciated. Inoculation wound completely healed, slight scab no caseous material or any signs of sputum Internal organs healthy; one white spot found on surface of liver. Microscopic examination of this showed it to consist of round cells, some with one nucleus and others which were polynuclear. At the periphery the nodule showed no tubercle bacilli.
B 4	Ditto in open watch-glass	July 10	Died Aug. 9	Emaciated, wound at back not healed, and appeared slightly sloughing at the borders. Lungs presented several small caseous nodules; pleura, heart, peritoneum, liver healthy. *Tubercle bacilli found in* the caseous lung nodules.

TABLE IV.—*Influence of Clay Soil, Bad Air, and Darkness*

No. of specimen.	Conditions of exposure.	Date of Inoculation.	Death.	Dr Dreschfeld's reports.
B 1	On dark shelf by fireplace in small cottage bedroom in Ancoats. Flask arrangement	June 27	Killed Sept. 4	Rabbit in good condition; wound completely healed, no caseation, and only a small pigmented spot where the sputum had been deposited; all the internal organs healthy.
B 5	Ditto in a dark corner near the bed. In watch-glass	July 10	Killed Sept. 4	Rabbit in good condition; cicatrix where the wound was, and beneath it a caseous mass about the size of a bean. Examined microscopically, this mass *contained tubercle bacilli.* Nothing abnormal in any of the organs.

TABLE V.—*Influence of Dry Soil, Bad Air, and Darkness*

No. of specimen.	Conditions of exposure.	Date of Inoculation.	Death.	Dr Dreschfeld's reports.
B 10	Cotton wool cage, in ventilating shaft from ward of Consumption Hospital for ten days, then placed on top of bookcase in sitting-room	July 10	Died Aug. 14	Emaciated; wound healed under a scab. A yellow caseous mass about the size of a small pea beneath the scab. The liver presented a few yellowish nodules; all the other organs sound. In the caseous mass *a few tubercle bacilli were found*; none in the liver.
B 10	A portion of the above was taken on the tenth day and exposed to a current of ozonised oxygen for a few minutes daily for a fortnight	July 10	Killed Sept. 4	Rabbit fairly well nourished; cicatrix quite healed, no trace of inoculated matter, and no trace of caseation. In the left lung one firm nodule; this was carefully examined microscopically and showed no bacilli. It was apparently only thickened pleura.

It will be seen that none of the four specimens of sputum exposed to fresh air and light on a dry soil conveyed the disease, but one of the three portions exposed under similar conditions in darkness produced tubercle.

Of the two exposed in the cottage in Ancoats in the light one produced tubercle, and of the two specimens exposed in the same place, in comparative darkness, one caused tubercle, the other did not.

Lastly, the specimen placed in the ventilating shaft from a ward in the Consumption Hospital, Bowdon, on a dry soil, conveyed the disease, and the portion removed from it after ten days and exposed to the action of ozonised oxygen did not produce tubercle.

These experiments are too few in number to justify the statement of positive conclusions, but, so far as they extend, they go to prove that fresh air and light and a dry sandy soil have a distinct influence in arresting the virulence of the tubercle bacillus ; that darkness somewhat interferes with this disinfectant action; and that the mere exposure to light in otherwise bad sanitary conditions does not destroy the virus. There are also some indications that the presence of a cotton wool envelope may interfere somewhat with the action for good or evil of both good and bad air respectively.

(5) ON RE-INFECTION IN PHTHISIS

MEDICAL CHRONICLE, *October*, 1892

THERE is ample proof of the existence in most large towns of tubercularly infected houses. I have called attention to some facts in support of this contention in a paper read before the Epidemiological Society in the year 1888, and the observations have been confirmed by Dr Niven, of Oldham, and Dr Tatham, of Manchester. Dr Flick, of Philadelphia, has also published an elaborate topographic study of phthisis in that city, which is conclusive on the point.

Dr Cornet's well-known researches are also of great importance in corroboration.

Hitherto, however, the existence of tubercular infection in houses has been considered chiefly as a source of danger to the healthy, but I wish to point out its importance to those who are, or have been, suffering from phthisis.

In his great work on *Traité de l'Auscultation Médiate* Laennec expresses (p. 699) the opinion that " no consumptive succumbs to a first attack of the tuberculous affection." He also gives his reasons for believing in the complete arrest of the disease in certain cases. The truth of the latter belief has now been abundantly proved, not only by the experience of all who have closely watched the progress of the disease, but also by the results of post-mortem examinations; and these last have the further advantage that they not only prove the possibility of cure, but demonstrate the very large proportion in which cures take place. Different observers give different proportions, varying from 50 per cent. (Cruveilhier, Rogée, Dégérini) to 26 per cent. (Standacker, Bollinger). The researches of Marsini and Dr Harris, of the Manchester Royal Infirmary, come near the mean at 39 per cent. of all the autopsies upon persons over twenty years of age who have died of other diseases than phthisis. It is natural that the figures should differ at different places owing to variations in the degree of infection, apart from differences of method, but it is obvious that in all places there must be a large number of persons in whom one attack at least had been recovered from, and who are unconscious of the peril through which they have passed.

In a very large number of cases, also, Laennec's first proposition is true, and we may extend it by saying that not only do they not die of the first attack, but not a few recover from it, and have no more seizures.

Unfortunately this occurrence is not so common amongst the patients of our consumptive hospitals as it is amongst the rich, or amongst those who can take the necessary precautions against further attacks.

This difference in the results naturally opens up another question—as to why, in so many cases, the patients suffer from a series of attacks until ultimately they end in death?—and again, whether there may not be something in the homes of the poorer class of patients that renders them more liable to a return of the disease?

The usual, and in many instances, the correct answer to this question is, that tuberculosis is an infective disease, that it spreads along the lymphatics or blood vessels, and that though the bacilli may cease for a time to irritate, and may many of them be discharged from the body, yet a sufficient number remain behind to sporulate and spread through the lungs or through the system, and this occurrence is most likely to occur in unhealthy conditions of life.

According to this theory, recovery takes place only because the tissues are so well nourished, or otherwise protected, that the bacilli cannot spread from their first focus, and at length are either entirely discharged or die out. If any subsequent attacks occur, this desirable result has not been obtained, but the bacilli or their spores have taken advantage of some temporary weakness or of some catarrh to make a fresh start into surrounding parts. As I have already acknowledged, this is probably a perfectly correct representation of the course of events in many cases.

But there is at least one other explanation of a revival of the disease, and that is by a *re-infection* from *external* sources, and if this occurrence is not rare, it points to a further source of danger to consumptive invalids.

It will no doubt be extremely difficult to prove in any given case that such re-infection has taken place, and that any particular outbreak of the disease has been due to such a cause, but a few considerations will show not only its possibility, but its extreme probability in a large number of cases.

(1) We have now the certainty that the primary infection must have come in most cases from external sources, and hence there can be nothing unusual in a second infection, or even in multiple infections, from similar surroundings.

(2) The patient has already proved himself to be susceptible of the disease, or vulnerable by the bacillus, and is therefore probably by nature more liable than others to the disease.

(3) By reason of his first attack also he is especially prone to become for a second time the host of the invading parasite. His damaged lung is less elastic, and less provided with the natural safeguards against its lodgement. We may also presume that the anti-microbic influences of the body, whether phagocytic or anti-toxic, are weaker than in the generality of human beings.

(4) It is almost certain that the primary source of infection was to be found in the unhealthy house, or in some usual haunt of the patient, and when he returns to his former condition of life he will probably meet with a contingent of the same enemy that made the first attack on his lungs.

(5) There is abundant evidence as to the existence of infected houses and infected workshops.

The distribution of phthisis in towns, and in places where bacillus-laden dust is most likely to be met with, its favourite haunts in badly ventilated, badly drained tenements, the evidence that now exists of the introduction of infection into houses, the discovery of the organism in these houses, and in places inhabited by consumptives—all these facts show the presence of the poison in the places from which most of our patients in hospital come, and make it most probable that the inhalation of the bacillus will take place again and again, and that it will be received into susceptible lungs.

(6) Under this head also we may note the longevity of the bacillus of tubercle in the presence of respiratory impurity— polluted ground air or other organic filth. If it does not gain in virulence under these circumstances (a not improbable event),

at least it is kept alive for long periods ; and the presence of a former consumptive, and the probability of his having left the specific poison somewhere in the house, make it still more likely that his home is a source of infection.

(7) And lastly, we come to the experience of individual medical men ; and although for the reasons already given, it will be impossible to affirm that re-infection, *ab extrâ*, has taken place in any one case, a frequent repetition of cases open to this interpretation will enhance the probability that some of them at least are of this character.

These considerations make the case for re-infection very strong. There are few hospital physicians who have not suffered the disappointment of seeing cases of phthisis deteriorate rapidly upon their return home, after they had greatly improved in hospital and had even shown signs of cure.

It is one of the most disheartening facts connected with the treatment of this disease in hospital, whatever may be the nature of the medicinal treatment. In the hospital, after the first two or three weeks, most of the cases begin to improve, fever diminishes, the cough and expectoration subside, and the patients gain weight, sometimes to a considerable extent. But when they are discharged, after a few weeks or months of residence, and are obliged to return to their former occupations or to their old homes, they frequently break down, and come back to the outdoor department with a fresh development of the disease.

This is a common experience at most consumptive hospitals, and it is, of course, open to the explanation that the fresh air and good food and healthy surroundings of the hospital kept the enemy at bay for the time ; but that it again advanced when the poor food and unhealthy conditions of the dwelling had so far lowered the patient's vital power that he could no longer resist its attacks.

No one can affirm that such a course as this is not in accordance with what we know of the natural progress of the disease ; and yet, from the considerations which have just been noted, it is at least as likely that the virus, instead of coming from within the body, has been derived from the poisonous atmosphere of the home. And in some of these cases there are certain facts to be noted that make the latter the most probable explanation of the case. Thus :

(1) In not a few instances, the disease, instead of spreading in a natural and usual fashion along the track of the absorbents, commences afresh in some part of the opposite lung, or in the larynx.

(2) In other instances the patient does not return home at once after leaving the hospital, but goes to stay with friends in the country, with people who are as poorly off as himself, where the main difference between his own home, and the place of his temporary sojourn, is fresh country air, and whilst he is under these otherwise unfavourable conditions, he still continues well and gains in weight, but after he finally returns home and has remained there only a few weeks, the disease again breaks out, makes rapid progress and soon comes to a fatal end.

(3) In some of the cases the interval between the first return home and the fresh outbreak of the disease is from three to six weeks, just about the usual incubation period of tubercular infection.

(4) Lastly, it is fair to count the numerous cases now known to have remained free from fresh outbreaks after change of residence, as, for the most part, instances of escape from re-infection from without. If, as some physicians contend, after a first attack the disease remains latent, waiting only for an opportunity to develop, it is difficult to understand why so many of these cases escape, in spite of the many depressing circumstances that often attend the change of residence and change of occupation.

It is precisely among those persons who take to a hard life, with exposure to out-door influences, often with poor and insufficient food, that we find our best instances of permanent cure. In many cases, in order to avoid the foul air, which I and so many others consider the chief source of danger, our poor patients often have to descend into a lower grade of labour, such as agricultural employment, omnibus conducting, ship stewardship, and so on, and yet the so-called latent tubercle finds no fresh point of attack, and the disease only re-appears when the patient has been exposed to new sources of infection from without. To my mind, the theory of re-development of latent tubercle

under these circumstances is contrary to all the canons of scientific
evidence.

The following cases will illustrate one or more of these points
tending to incriminate the infected home.

Case 1.—J. T. J., æt. 19, was admitted to the hospital on
January 10, 1888, with softening tubercle at the right apex, and
slight consolidation on the left side. His weight on admission
was 108 lbs., and under treatment by iodoform, cod-liver oil,
and ozone inhalations (five cylinders daily), he improved steadily,
the disease remaining absolutely stationary, though bacilli were
abundant in the sputum. He was discharged on April 27,
weighing 124¾ lbs.—a gain of more than 16 lbs. He then went
to stay with friends at a little farm in Wales, where the food was
scanty, but he continued to improve, and gained 10 lbs. more in
weight in the course of this year and the next. He returned to
his own home in the autumn of 1889, and he was re-admitted to
the hospital on November 22, 1889. He still looked robust and
well, and weighed 135 lbs. His left lung was normal, and there
were no signs of extension of disease on the right side, but his
voice was hoarse, and on laryngoscopic examination tubercular
infiltration of the epiglottis was found to be commencing. From
this time he steadily lost ground, the disease spreading through
the right lung and in the larynx, and he died in the spring of
1891.

Case 2.—E. F., male, æt. 29, was admitted to hospital on
July 18, 1888, with a twelve months' history of phthisis, now in
the second stage on the left side and slight consolidation at the
right apex. His weight on admission was 141½ lbs., and after
four months' treatment with cod-liver oil and ozone inhalations
he gained 5¼ lbs. in weight, and the disease in the lungs remained
stationary. He was discharged on November 5, but was re-
admitted on January 18, 1889, having lost 10 lbs. in weight,
and with an extension of disease in the right lung and a cavity
in the apex. He regained 7 lbs. in weight in the next two months,
and improved for a time, but after his discharge he again rapidly
lost ground and died in the autumn.

Case 3.—R. H., male, æt. 17, admitted May 5, 1889, had
hæmoptysis six months before—now a cavity in the right apex—

left side normal. He was treated with iodoform, cod-liver oil, and ozone inhalations (three cylinders thrice daily), and on September 10 he was discharged, having gained 6 lbs. in weight, and with the note that " the disease had not progressed in the slightest." He returned home, but was re-admitted on November 19, having lost 7 lbs. in weight, with softening tubercle on the left side, considerable extension of the disease on the right, and with tubercular laryngitis. He died a few months later.

Case 4.—J. B., male, æt. 29, clerk, admitted to hospital April 17, 1885, with softening tubercle at both apices (one year's history). He remained five weeks, taking chiefly iodoform and cod-liver oil, and improved very much, gaining several pounds in weight. He then (in June, 1885) went to Canada, but returned in fourteen months. He had been employed as a farm labourer, and found the food inferior and the hardship great, but notwithstanding this, he had gained weight, and the disease had not advanced in the least. In September, 1886, he went home, and in March, 1887, he was re-admitted as an in-patient, with increased disease on the right side. He again improved, however, and left in June, weighing 121 lbs. He returned to work and to his old home, and in April, 1889, he was again received as an in-patient, having lost 19 lbs. in weight, and with a large vomica in the left upper lobe.

Case 5.—A. W., female, æt. 16, weaver, had hæmoptysis in September, 1890, and twice in the spring of 1891. Was admitted to hospital on May 20, 1891, with a vomica at the left apex and slight consolidation of the right. Sputum crowded with bacilli (B. 3). She was treated with creasote and cod-liver oil and carbolic inhalation, afterwards with iodoform, and was discharged on December 11, having gained 20 lbs. in weight. The cavity contracting, the sputum much diminished in quantity and the bacilli reduced to B. 1.

A place as waiting-maid was found for her in the country, but before going to it she went home to Bradford, in Manchester, for a week. Three weeks after going to her situation she fell ill, with increased cough and expectoration, fever, and night sweats, which lasted several weeks. Three months after her recovery she came to the out-patient department and was examined, and although the disease was again quiescent, it was evident that there had been an extension of the disease in the right lung.

Case 6.—S. D., boxmaker. Phthisical history of three years. Admitted to hospital May 13, 1889, with large cavity in right apex. Left side, doubtful consolidation at apex. In three months gained 21 lbs. in weight on cod-liver oil and iodoform. Returned home, and to work six or seven hours a day. Cough returned three months later, and she lost 13 lbs. in weight.

Re-admitted October 4, 1890, with softening tubercle in the left upper lobe ; no extension of the disease on the right side. She died in the spring of 1892.

Cases of Phthisis who had Changed their Residence

No.	Name	Sex	Age	Stage	Duration of Life		
1	McK.	Male	34	Third	Living	7	years after
2	Mrs C.	Female	35	First	Died	20	,,
3	L. C.	,,	30	,,	Living	26	,,
4	Miss R.	,,	25	,,	,,	15	,,
5	Mrs J.	,,	30	Second	,,	20	,,
6	G. S.	,,	18	First	,,	17	,,
7	Th. J.	Male	45	,,	,.	20	,,
8	F. R.	,,	36	,,	,,	14	,,
9	W. W.	,,	45	,,	,,	10	,,
10	Mrs M. W.	Female	25	Third	,,	17	,,
11	,, K.	,,	39	Second	,,	12	,,
12	,, S.	,,	30	First	,,	20	,,
13	,, D.	,,	30	,,	,,	18	,,
14	J. G.	Male	28	Second	,,	40	,,
15	A. B.	,,	19	First	,,	20	,,
16	F. G.	,,	18	,,	,,	18	,,
17	C. C.	,,	47	Second	,,	30	,,
18	A. H.	Female	18	First	,,	20	,,
19	D. W.	Male	30	Third	Died	40	,,
20	H. B.	Female	20	Second	Living	8	,,

These cases are not to be regarded in any sense statistically. They are merely examples of a numerous series of instances of similar character which have come under my notice at the Manchester Hospital for Consumption. Not one of these detailed cases can be recorded as a distinct and undoubted instance of re-infection, for in each there is the possibility that the subsequent outburst of disease had an internal source ; but the repeated occurrence of such cases, viewed in the light of the *a priori* considerations which have been mentioned, has left a profound impression on my own mind, and has led me to affirm the strong probability of re-infection upon a patient's return to previous conditions of life.

It also leads to the enquiry as to the best means of preventing such an occurrence, especially in the numerous class of cases in which removal to another dwelling cannot be carried out, and I venture to think that the practical lessons to be drawn from the facts are : (1) the need either of change of residence, or of the thorough disinfection of premises occupied or frequented by consumptive persons ; (2) the duty of constantly destroying by fire or corrosive sublimate the sputum from these patients.

These measures have hitherto been chiefly advocated on the plea that they are necessary for the protection of other members of the family or of the public ; but if it be true that in many cases of phthisis the primary lesions would entirely heal unless fresh infection takes place, it becomes a part of our treatment for the cure of these cases to take care that these measures are carried out.

It may be stated that these considerations have so far weighed with the Medical Officers of Health for Manchester and Salford, Drs Tatham and Paget, that they have agreed to disinfect any houses notified to them by the medical staff of the Hospital for Consumption, and this course has already been carried out in several instances in the Manchester district. Experiments as to the most efficient system of disinfection are also being carried out, under the direction of Professor Delépine, of the Owens College.

(6) ON CERTAIN MEDIA FOR THE CULTIVATION OF THE BACILLUS OF TUBERCLE[1]

In May, 1894, a communication was made to the Society by Professor Delépine and myself, " On the Influence of certain Natural Agents on the Virulence of the Tubercle-Bacillus." The conclusions drawn from the experiments recorded in this paper were :

(1) That finely divided tuberculous matter, such as pure cultures of the bacillus, or tuberculous matter derived from sputum, in daylight and in free currents of air is rapidly deprived of virulence ;

(2) That even in the dark, although the action is retarded, fresh air has still some disinfecting influence ; and

(3) That in the absence of air, or in confined air, the bacillus retains its power for long periods of time.

These observations afforded an explanation of the immunity of certain places, and the danger of infection in others. They show that where tuberculous sputum is exposed to sufficient light and air, to deprive it of virulence before it can be dried up and powdered into dust, no danger of infection need be dreaded. It would appear further, from this research and others, that it is only when there is sufficient organic material in the air, derived from impure ground air, or from the reek of human bodies, that the tubercle bacillus can retain its existence and its virulent power. Long-lived though it may be under these latter conditions, it is rapidly disinfected by the natural agencies of fresh air and sunlight ; so rapidly that, when these agents are present, even in comparatively moderate degree, the tuberculous material cannot reach its dangerous state of dust before it is deprived of all power of doing harm.

[1] By permission of the Royal College of Physicians, this research, which forms a portion of the Weber-Parkes Prize Essay, is communicated to the Royal Society before publication. The cost of the inquiry is defrayed by the Thrustan prize, presented to the author this year by Gonville and Caius College, Cambridge.

But, in addition to the above-mentioned researches, it seemed desirable that an attempt should be made to ascertain what part was played respectively by the several forms of organic impurity that are present in insanitary dwellings. Hitherto, so far as I know, no attempt has been made, in the laboratory or elsewhere, to imitate the actual conditions that prevail in such houses. It was determined, therefore, to collect the aqueous vapours arising from the ground or from human bodies, and to submit these products to the test of trying whether they would serve as cultivating media for the bacillus of tubercle.

Many years ago in a research, the particulars of which are given in an appendix to my treatise on " Stethometry," I examined the condensed aqueous vapour of the breath, in health and disease, and ascertained the quantity of organic matter that it contained. The breath of 15 healthy persons and of 27 cases of disease was examined chemically by Wanklyn's method of water analysis, and microscopically. The fact of chief importance obtained was, that every specimen contained a small, but appreciable, quantity of both free and organic ammonia. The quantity from the cases of disease varied considerably, but that from healthy persons was remarkably constant, varying from 0·325 milligram to 0·45 per 100 minims of the fluid collected, 'the average being 0·4. Hence, by calculation, we obtain the rough estimate that about 3 grs. of organic matter is given off from a man's lungs in the course of 24 hours. Doubtless a very small amount, but sufficient to render the aqueous vapour thus thrown off more impure than most sewage water, and ample in quantity to foster the growth of organic germs.

It was the result of this research that induced me to try to cultivate the bacillus of tubercle upon these and similar organic fluids, such as were likely to be met with in dwelling-houses.

By means of a simple freezing mixture of ice and salt it was easy to condense the aqueous vapour, both of the breath and that coming from ground air ; and, in order to make the inquiry more complete, the vapour of the breath was collected in a flask, surrounded by this mixture, from both healthy and diseased sources. In other words, both healthy persons and those affected by phthisis were prevailed upon to breathe into the flask, until a sufficient quantity of aqueous fluid had been obtained. With another apparatus, consisting of a framework supporting beakers containing freezing mixture, collections of aqueous fluid were obtained from " ground air " coming from a wine cellar in a gravelly subsoil, and from cellars under several low-lying, insanitary cottages in Southampton. Some of the moisture from a weaving-shed in Blackburn was also thus collected and used as a cultivating medium. The composition of these latter fluids is given below :

TABLE I.—*Composition of condensed Aqueous Vapours from following sources*

Sources of fluids	Parts of weight of ammonias per 100,000		Grains per gallon of ammonias	
	Free and saline	Albuminoid	Free and saline	Albuminoid
Healthy breath	1·622	3·568	1·135	2·497
Phthisical breath ..	0·973	2·598	0·681	1·816
Bournemouth cellar air	0·649	1·622	0·454	1·135
Southampton cellar air	2·141	3·893	1·498	2·724
Pure sandy soil	0·020	0·030		
Blackburn weaving sheds (average) (humidified)	0·319	0·082	0·223	0·057
Thames sewage at South Outfall (Keats) ..	2·309	3·893	1·498	2·724

These several liquids were carefully sterilised by repeated boilings, and were then used, in various ways, for the cultivation of the bacillus of tubercle[1].

Two well-grown specimens of pure cultivations were obtained (both through Dr Childs), one (A) from the Institute of Preventive Medicine, the other (B) from a private source, but the latter specimen could not be guaranteed as human bacillus, it was therefore labelled as of doubtful origin, and the cultivations made with it were kept separate.

In order to test the activity of these cultures they were each, in the first instance, sown upon (a) sterilised blood serum, and

[1] The various manipulations involved in this inquiry were carried out chiefly by Mr Tanner, in his Bacteriological Laboratory, at Bournemouth and to his carefulness and skill much of the success attained is due

(*b*) upon "glycerine agar peptone," as these media were known to be the best for cultivating purposes, and the results could then with advantage be compared with those from the other materials used.

Both specimens were found to be capable of active growth, though the cultivation (A) was somewhat tardy.

TABLE II

Media		Date of inocula-tion	Periods of incubation (at 35° C.)			
			2 weeks	4 weeks	8 weeks	12 weeks and upwards.
Blood serum	A	April 3	..	×	× ×	× × ×
Agar peptone	A	,, ,,	..	×	× ×	× × ×
Blood serum	B	,, ,,	× ×	× × ×	× × ×	
Glycerine agar	B	,, 13	×	× ×	× × ×	× × ×
Agar peptone	B	,, 3	× ×	× × ×	× × ×	

The crosses denote degrees of growth. One × means the first appearance of a colony. Two × ×, two or more colonies, evidently growing. Three × × ×, growth extending over medium.

It was then thought well, in the first instance, to attempt to cultivate the bacillus upon media on which it grows with difficulty, without the presence of added peptones ; in other words, to find out whether the presence of the condensed organic fluids from the sources that have been mentioned would replace the peptones.

Accordingly, simple agar jelly, with 5 per cent. of glycerine, was made with each of the fluids mentioned, after careful sterilisation. Tubes were charged with these several compounds, inoculated with looped platinum wire lightly charged, stoppered with sterilised wool, capped, and placed in an incubator, kept at a temperature of 35° C. At the same time, slips of potato, after thorough sterilisation, were soaked in the fluids and inoculated and similarly disposed of.

As a control experiment, the agar jelly was made with simple distilled water and glycerine, charged and disposed of in the same way.

The results of these several experiments are shown on the two following tables. It will be observed that, out of the 18 specimens, only two (two of those from the impure cellars) failed to produce growth to some extent; those that did best were the fluids from the cellar in porous soil, and those condensed from the breath of phthisical patients. But all kinds of organic fluid showed growth on either agar jelly or potato.

TABLE III

No.		Date of inocula-tion	Periods of incubation and growth (in incubator at 35° C.)			
			2 weeks	4 weeks	8 weeks	12 weeks and upwards
	Media : Agar c̄ 5 per cent. glycerine	April 13	..	×	× ×	× ×
	Condensed vapour from the following sources :					
1	Cellar in pure porous soil ..	April 3	×	× ×	× × ×	× × ×
2	Ditto	,, ,,	×	× ×	× × ×	× × × ×
3	Ditto	,, 10	..	..	×	faint
4	Ditto	,, ,,	..	..	×	,,
5	Impure cellar on clay	,, ,,	..	..	..	blank
6	Ditto	,, ,,	..	..	..	,,
7	Healthy breath	,, ,,	..	×	×	× ×
8	Ditto	,, ,,	..	×	×	× ×
9	Phthisical breath	,, 3	×	× ×	× × ×	× × × blackened
10	Ditto	,, ,,	×	× ×	× × ×	× × × blackened

There is thus some evidence that the organic fluids facilitated cultivation to some extent; experienced bacteriologists, who have attempted to use simple potato or glycerine agar as the cultivating medium, have assured me that failure is much more common than success, and that the growth, when it does take place, is usually very slow. With the organic fluids there were only two failures, and growth was fairly rapid.

In the next series of trials, it was decided to use as the material bases some non-nitrogenous substance, and attempts were made to employ pieces of wood, cork, cotton-wool, and fine spun glass, the last named at the suggestion of a distinguished bacteriologist. None of these bases was found to be satisfactory; and at length

TABLE IV

No.		Date of inocula-tion	Periods of incubation and growth (in incubator at 35° C.)			
			2 weeks	4 weeks	8 weeks	12 weeks and upwards
	Media : Sterilised potato,and the vapours as above					
1	From cellar in pure porous soil	April 3	×	× × ×	× × × ×	× × × ×
2	Ditto	,, ,,	×	× ×	× ×	feeble
3	Impure cellar in clay	,, 10	..	..	× ×	× × ×
4	Ditto	,, ,,	..	..	× ×	× × ×
5	Healthy breath	,, ,,	..	×	× ×	× ×
6	Ditto	,, ,,	..	× ×	× ×	× × ×
7	Phthisical breath	,, 3	..	×	× ×	× × ×

it was determined to use a particularly pure "filter-paper," manufactured by Messrs Schleicher and Schüll, from which even the salts had been extracted by washing with hydrochloric and hydrofluoric acids[1]. This paper was folded in a convenient form, sterilised, inserted in the test-tubes, and charged with the several organic fluids, to which, as before, 6 per cent. of pure glycerine had been added. It was then inoculated, stoppered as before, and in the first trials these tubes were placed in the incubator at the usual temperature of 35° C.

The results are shown on Table V.

It will be seen that some degree of success was attained in 12 out of 15 specimens of the organic fluids. The degree of growth was also much the same as in the previous series, though perhaps slightly less vigorous.

It was now determined to try to do without the help of the glycerine, which, as is well known, so greatly assists the ordinary cultivations of the bacillus. Accordingly, four tubes with simple filter-paper as the supporting medium, and condensed fluids, from the breath of a healthy person, and from that of a phthisical patient, as nutrient fluids, were inoculated, and no glycerine was

[1] Each of these filter-papers, analysed for me by the Kjeldahl process, by Sir H. Roscoe's assistant, was found to contain only 0·1 milligram of nitrogen.

TABLE V

No.	Media: Chemically pure filter-paper and condensed fluids 5 per cent. glycerine	Date of inoculation	Periods of cultivation (in incubator at 35° C.)				Remarks
			2 weeks	4 weeks	8 weeks	12 weeks	
	Culture A						
1	From pure cellar air ..	May 23	..	×	××	××	
2	,, ,, impure ..	,, ,,	..	×	×	××	
3	,, impure cellar air	,, ,,	×		××	×××	
4	,, ,,	June 5	×	××	××	×	
5	,, weaver's shed	,, ,,	..	×	×	××	
6	,, ,,	,, ,,	..	×	××	×××	
7	,, healthy breath	,, ,,	..	×	××	×××	
8	,, ,,	,, ,,	..	×	××	×××	
9	,, phthisical breath	May 23	×	×	××	×××	
10	,, ,,	,, ,,					
11	Distilled water ,,	,, ,,	..	..	..	..	Medium found to contain free ammonia
12	,, ,,	,, ,,	..	?	..	..	
	Culture B						
1	Pure cellar air	,, ,,	?	×	××	××	
2	Impure ditto ..	,, ,,					
3	Weaver's shed	June 5	?	××	×	××	
4	Healthy breath	May 23	?	××	××	×××	
5	Phthisical breath	,, ,,					
6	Distilled water	,, ,,					

added. In these tubes the same cultivation was used as in the previous experiments.

Shortly afterwards, two similar tubes with fluid from healthy breath alone, but with 5 per cent. of glycerine, were sown with the same cultivation, and were left at the ordinary temperature of the laboratory, about 21° C. (see Table VI).

All of the former group took on active growth within four weeks, and one of the latter. In other words, it was proved that pure filter-paper, moistened with these condensed fluids alone, would suffice to nourish and promote the growth of the bacillus, and, further, that this growth would take place at ordinary temperatures. It may hence be concluded that when this organic fluid is present in ordinary dwellings, the bacillus may grow at the temperature of living rooms as well as at the temperature of 35° C.

In September, 1896, another attempt to test this point was made by inoculating a dozen more tubes in which the various condensed fluids were employed as nutrients. Some of them were placed in the incubator, the others being placed outside.

In this series, however, a sub-culture on agar peptone, taken from the old Preventive Institute tube, was used as the seed ; and it was soon evident that this sub-culture had greatly declined in vigour. For three months no perceptible growth took place on any of the specimens, and then only on phthisical breath to a very slight extent. Although they must be counted for the most part as failures, the results of the inoculations are given in Table VI.

In consequence of this failure in vigour of the last used cultivation, a fresh series of eight tubes was commenced on October 31 with the same cultivation, which also failed.

Then, in February, 1897, through the kindness of Dr Childs and of Dr Curtis, a fresh tube of apparently vigorous cultivation of the tubercle bacillus, guaranteed to be of human origin, was obtained from University College, London.

By way of control, this culture was sown upon blood serum and upon agar peptone, and incubated at 37° C., and a copious growth was found to be commencing on the blood serum within ten days' time (see Table IX).

Two sets of tubes were then prepared of condensed vapour from breath, and from ground air from a pure sandy soil. No

TABLE VI

No.	Date of inoculation	Periods of cultivation				
		2 weeks	4 weeks	8 weeks	12 weeks	16 weeks
	Media: Pure filter-paper with condensed fluids alone (no glycerine).					
	Culture A					
	In incubator at 35° C.					
1	Healthy breath July 21	..	×	× ×	× ×	
2	,, ,, ,,	..	×	×	×	
3	Phthisical breath ,,	..	×	×	×	
4	,, ,, ,,	×	× ×	× × ×	× × ×	
	Ditto with 5 per cent. glycerine at temperature of laboratory (or about 21° C.)					
1	Healthy breath ,,					
2	,, ,, ,,	×	× ×	× ×	× ×	
	Sub-culture from A					
	Same medium, without glycerine	1 mnth	2 mnths	3 mnths	4 mnths	
1	Phthisical breath Sept. 17	..	..	..	×	×
2	Ditto, 35° C. ,,					
3	Ditto, ordinary temp. ,,					
4	Ditto, ordinary temp. ,,					
5	Healthy breath ,,					
6	Ditto, 35° C. ,,					
7	Ditto, ordinary temp. ,,					
8	Ditto, ordinary temp. ,,					
9	Blackburn shed, 35° C. Sept. 24					
10	Ditto, 35° C. ,,					
11	Ditto, ordinary temp.					
12	Ditto, ordinary temp.					

TABLE VII

No.	Media : Pure filter-paper, c̄ following vapours and ½ per cent. gelatine	Temperature	Date of inoculation	Periods of cultivation				Remarks
				2 weeks	4 weeks	2 months	3 months	
96	Pure ground air	37° C.	Feb. 10	x	x x	x x x	x x x	
97	,, ,,	,,	,,	x x	x	x x x	x x	
100	Healthy breath	,,	,,	x x	x	x	x x	
101	,, ,,	,,	,,				x x	
	Same, without gelatine							
104	Pure ground air	22	,,	x	x	x	x x	{ Removed from incubator 9th day
105	,,	37	,,	x x	x x	x x	x x x	
106	,,	,,	,,	x x	x x	x x	x x x	
122	,,	22	Mar. 2	...	x	x	x	Ditto
123	,,	,,	,,	x	x	x	x x	Ditto
124	,,	37	,,	x	x x	x x	sent away	
125	,,	,,	,,	x	x	x x	x x	
126	,,	,,	,,	x	x	x x	x x x	
127	,,	,,	,,	x	x x	x	x x x	
128	,,	22	,,	x	x	x x	x x x	
116	Healthy breath	22	,,	x	x x	x	x x x	
117	,, ,,	37	,,	x	x	x	x x	

TABLE VIII

No.	Media: Lining wall-paper, c̄ vapours and ½ per cent. gelatine	Temperature	Date of inoculation	Period of cultivation				Remarks
				2 weeks	4 weeks	2 months	3 months	
98	Pure ground air	37° C.	Feb. 10	x	x x	x x	x x	
99	,, ,,	,,	,,	x	x x	x x x	x x x	
102	Healthy breath	,,	,,	x x	x x	x x	x x	
103	,, ,,	,,	,,	x x	x x	x x	x x	
	Same, without gelatine							
108	Pure ground air	22	,,	x	x	x x	x x	{ Removed from incubator 9th day
107	,,	37	,,	x x	x x	x x	x x	
109	,,	,,	,,	x x	x x	x x x	x x	
110	,,	,,	,,	x x x	x x	x x	x x	
111	,,	,,22	,,	x x x	x x x	x x	x x	
112	,,	,,	Mar. 2	x x	x x	x x	x x	Ditto
129	,,	,,	,,	x	x x	x x	sent away	
130	,,	,,	,,	x x	x x	x x	x x	
134	,, ,,	37	,,	x x	x x x	x x x	x x x	
119	Healthy breath	,,	,,	x x	x x	x x	x x	
121	,,	,,22	,,	: x	x	x	x x	
118	,,	,,	,,	x	x	x x	x x	
120	,, ,,	37	,,	x x	x x x	x x	x x	
131	Pure ground air	,,	,,	x x	x x	x x x	x x x	
132	,,	,,	,,	x x	x x	x x	x x	
133	,,	,,	,,	x	x x	x x	x x x	
135	,,	,,	,,	x	x x	x	x x	

TABLE IX.—*Control Cultivations*

No.	Media	Temperature	Date of inoculation	Periods of cultivation				Remarks
				2 weeks	4 weeks	2 months	3 months	
113	Blood serum	37° C.	Feb. 10	x	x x x	x x x	x x x	
114	Agar peptone	,,	,,	x	x x	x x x	x x x	
136	Blood serum	,,	Mar. 2	·	x x x	x x x x x	x x	
137	,,	22	,,	x	·		x x	
138	Agar peptone	37	,,	x	x x	x x	x x x	
139	,,	22	,,	·	x	x	x x	
140	Gelatine peptone	,,	,,					
141	,,	,,	,,					
142	Potato tubes	37	,,	x ?	x x	x x	x x x	
143	,,	,,	,,	x	x	x x	x x x	
144	,,	22	,,	·		x	x	
145	,,	,,	,,	·				

glycerine was added ; but for the solid medium, in some instances, the pure filter-paper was employed ; in others, an ordinary lining paper, containing a little size, but carefully sterilised, was used.

Some of these were placed in the incubator at a temperature of 37° C., as this higher degree was thought more favourable to growth ; others were left in the dark at the ordinary temperature of the laboratory. The results are shown on Tables VII and VIII.

It will be seen that in many of the tubes a free growth was observed as early as the end of the first fortnight.

Out of the total number in this series of 37, in 36 instances there was free growth on the medium employed, on both kinds of paper, and all kinds of condensed fluid. Eleven of them were grown at a temperature of about 20° C. In only one instance was there complete failure (vapour from healthy breath).

Most of these tubes have been left intact, in order that they may be inspected ; but six of them were removed, stained, and examined microscopically, in order to determine whether they were true cultures ; this they proved to be.

Two of the cultures, after two months' growth, were sent away to be inoculated into guinea-pigs, but both they and the original culture were found to be non-virulent.

Microscopic Examination

Nearly all the earlier cultures, in which there appeared to have been any growth, were submitted to microscopical examination. In all the specimens in which this examination did not show distinct signs of growth the result was put down as " nil," even though a small number of bacilli might have been found. These few bacilli might have come from the inoculation. It was not difficult to recognise the abundant growth of a true cultivation.

These examinations, however, gave remarkable results in a large number of the specimens grown upon paper. Many of the bacilli were gigantic in size, and a considerable number of them showed distinct branching. Others were knobbed at one end or at both ends, when they looked like miniature " life pre-servers." In many of the specimens the culture seemed to have penetrated into the substance of the paper. (See Micro-photograph opposite.)

The bearing of these researches upon the subject of the pro-phylaxis against tuberculosis seems to be of some importance.

They prove that any one of the various organically charged vapours, whether coming from healthy or from diseased lungs, from the air of cellars, or from comparatively pure ground, forms an excellent cultivating medium for the bacillus of tubercle when kept away from the disinfecting influence of air and light.

This power of promoting its growth is particularly manifest when the supporting substance is common wall-paper, though it is quite apparent when very pure filter-paper is used.

It is further proved that, on these substances, the growth of the bacillus may take place at the ordinary temperatures of dwelling-rooms ; and, hence, that there is no safety against the increase of the organism in ordinary living rooms in which active tuberculous dust is present, and in which the natural disinfectants of the bacillus, fresh air and light, are not present in sufficient amount to destroy their virulence.

Plate I

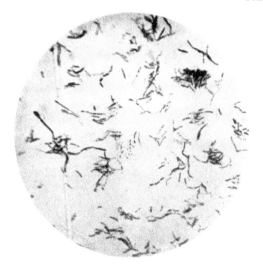

Micro-photograph (by Dr Dixon) of culture of B.T. on wall-paper, moistened by aqueous vapour of human breath, at ordinary summer temperature. (The tuberculous material was supplied by Dr C. Childs from a human joint in University College Hospital.)

(7) THE TUBERCLE BACILLUS AS A SAPROPHYTE

As an outcome of some of his earliest researches, Dr Koch pronounced the tubercle bacillus to be a true parasite, which can only originate in an animal organism. In a paper, "The Etiology of Tuberculosis," published in 1884, he emphasised this conclusion, on the grounds that "experience has shown that tubercle-bacilli grow much more slowly than any other bacteria, further that they grow only in serum and meat infusion, and most important of all, require a temperature of 30° C. to grow at all." He repeats "they are therefore true parasites which cannot live without their host."

It was not long before this conclusion was challenged by Mr Candler, of Melbourne, mainly on the ground of insufficient proof[1], and shortly afterwards several bacteriologists, foremost among whom were Sir Hugh Beevor, the late Prof. Kanthack, and Prof. Delépine, succeeded in cultivating the organism, not only on a variety of purely vegetable substances, but even at temperatures much below that of the animal body, 15° C. and under.

I have myself been able to grow the bacillus at ordinary temperatures, and have obtained abundant colonies on such simple media as pure filter-paper, common wall-paper, and potato, moistened with watery fluids obtained by condensing the vapours from human breath, from ground air, and from weaving sheds.

It is still a question whether these non-parasitic cultures retain sufficient virulence to give the disease to animals, but apart from direct evidence, I think that there are several considerations which point to the conclusion that they are a source of danger in this respect.

In the first place, it is certain that tuberculous sputum retains its vitality and its virulence for very long periods of time, when exposed in low-lying, badly-drained dwellings, inhabited by a densely-packed population, and that it rapidly loses its power in well-lighted, well-drained houses, placed on a dry, porous subsoil.

[1] *The Prevention of Consumption.*

I venture to refer to some experiments on this point, made in collaboration with Professor Dreschfeld, of Manchester, and reported in the *Proceedings of the Royal Society*[1].

I have further proved, by an inquiry into the incidence of tubercular disease in certain parts of Manchester and Salford, that the complaint clings to infected houses situated in these districts[2].

Dr Flick, of Philadelphia, also showed that phthisis has a special affinity for particular groups of houses, in which it keeps recurring : and Dr Niven found the same distribution of the disease in Oldham. More recently the Public Health Department in the city of New York has plotted out the cases occurring on a series of maps, and it is thus seen that houses are affected in blocks, and are passed over in blocks. In fact, it looks as if one house affected another, rather than that one person affected another.

It seems probable from these results that these unhealthy houses contained something which is at least favourable to the existence of the microbe, and that this material sufficed both to nourish it and facilitate its growth.

The special experiments which I have already mentioned show that the condensed organic vapours commonly found in such houses form admirable cultivating media for the growth of the bacillus.

I venture to think that these facts prove that the bacillus of tubercle is not merely a parasite, but that it can live upon material outside the body, and they point to the probable nature of this material.

In any case there can be no doubt that the organism can nourish itself, at ordinary temperatures, upon substances commonly met with in dwellings ; upon the aqueous vapour contained in the breath of human beings, or proceeding from the soil.

To this extent, therefore, the bacillus of tubercle is a " saprophyte."

Some other researches, carried out in 1894, in collaboration with Prof. Delépine[3], still further explain the immunity of certain houses, and infection in others, and indicate other sources of

---

[1] Vol. xlix. p. 66. [2] *Trans. of Epid. Soc. of London*, vol. vi, N.S.
[3] *Proc. R. S.* vol. lvi.

danger in unwholesome dwellings. In these researches we were able to prove that the virulence of tuberculous sputum is rapidly destroyed by exposure to pure air and sunlight ; so rapidly that it has not time to dry up, and crumble into dust, before it has entirely lost its virulence.

The practical lessons to be learnt from these several series of facts are, I venture to think, (1) that local authorities must seek out all the phthisis nests in their districts, and either purify them effectually or destroy them ; (2) that they must wage war against overcrowding and imperfect ventilation of dwellings, workshops, and places of public assembly ; (3) that they must carefully carry out subsoil drainage, and must insist upon concrete basements, and damp-courses in all buildings.

These measures are of no less importance than the disinfection of sputum, or the segregation of careless people in Sanatoria, or even than the formation of herds of tubercle-free cattle. All this should be done, but the other general sanitary work should not be left undone.

SECTION IV. CHIEFLY STATISTICAL

(1) SOME EVIDENCE RESPECTING TUBERCULAR INFECTIVE AREAS

Reprinted from the Transactions of the Epidemiological Society of London, Vol. vi, n.s., 1888

THERE are strong reasons for believing that whilst tubercle travels infectively through the body, and is derived from infective particles contained in air rendered impure by respiration, yet in this climate that it is very rarely produced by direct infection from person to person. It seems most probable, in fact, that for the active propagation of the disease, some increase in the virulence of the organism must take place outside the body, this intensification of its power being most commonly produced by the presence of animal organic matter in the air, in other words, by the absence of efficient ventilation. The favouring influence of a damp subsoil is also very distinct, and is probably due to the quality of the ground air arising from such soil. With such premises as these it might fairly be anticipated that certain distinct areas of infection would be found in both town and country, though most abundantly in crowded, ill-ventilated houses in the low-lying, badly-drained districts of towns.

Perhaps the best examples of infective areas are to be found in the records of public institutions, such as workhouses, prisons, orphanages, etc. Hirsch, in his *Handbook of Geographical Pathology*[1], gives a long list of such instances relating to scrofula, and others relating to consumption in vol. iii. p. 222.

Dr Parkes, also, in his work on Hygiene[2], gives some additional examples ; and Laennec, in his classical treatise on Phthisis, records one notable instance of the kind, in which the population

[1] *Syd. Soc.* vol. ii. p. 632.   [2] 6th ed. p. 134.

of a religious community of women had been changed two or three times from phthisis, with the notable exception of those who had charge of the garden, kitchen, and infirmary. The records of death from phthisis in the army, from unhealthy barracks, in all quarters of the globe, and similar returns from unhealthy ships in the navy, and in the mercantile marine, show the same thing. I believe all these accounts to be instances of bacillary infection from the fostering influence of bad air or bad drainage, or both.

But if the theory is sound, it ought to be possible also to find examples of breeding-places for the disease, "phthisis nests" as they might be called, in the narrow streets and courts, and even in individual houses in our towns.

The inquiry is one of some difficulty. It is thus not always possible to separate the effects of hereditary tendency to the disease from those of unhealthy areas, and the question of the possibility of direct contagion also enters the arena of discussion. With regard to the first-mentioned source of difficulty, however, it must be remarked that, according to our present knowledge of the matter, a hereditary tendency to consumption, or the scrofulous diathesis, as it used to be called, means little more than a peculiar vulnerability of the system by the specific organism, and hence it simply intensifies the operation of favouring external circumstances. It will thus assist both direct and indirect infection.

The possibility and probability of the direct conveyance of the disease, from patient to patient, is of more importance in regard to our immediate subject, seeing that many of the cases supposed to be due to local conditions and indirect infection might just as reasonably be ascribed to direct infection. I would also grant at once that there is nothing antecedently improbable in the theory of direct infection, although such infection would be likely to be difficult to persons in a healthy condition.

Professor Koch has shown that the bacillus of tubercle needs for its development: (1) a suitable medium containing organic matter, such as ox-blood serum, or the Japanese gelatinous substance, agar-agar; (2) a temperature of between 87° and 106°; (3) a sojourn of a week or more under these conditions.

It is probable that the last-named condition accounts for the immunity of the healthy lung to its attacks. The bacillus can obtain ready access to the air-passages of us all, seeing that it is probably often contained in the dusty atmosphere of towns or in the impure air of meetings at which some consumptive or other may be present. It would also find both suitable pabulum and a suitable temperature within the human thorax, but from healthy lungs it would soon be ejected, either entangled in mucus, or passed out by the action of the cilia lining the air-tubes. Such a fate need not necessarily befall it, however, if the lung had lost its natural elasticity by cramped and confined positions of the body, or by attacks of inflammation of the substance of the lung ; and we know that such attacks are common precursors of true phthisis. There would be nothing wonderful, therefore, in the direct engrafting of tubercle upon such lungs, and yet I believe that such direct transference of the disease from one person to another is a very rare event in this climate.

I have elsewhere given my reasons for coming to this conclusion, but I may perhaps be allowed to give their substance here.

1. We may note, as the result of a special inquiry conducted by the Collective Investigation Committee of the British Medical Association, extending over a period of many years, that, out of some millions of cases of phthisis that must have occurred during this time, there are only a few hundreds of supposed cases of infection deemed worthy of record, and many medical men expressly state that they have never seen a case of direct infection.

2. Upon analysing these cases by means of Dr Longstaff's formula, given in the *Collective Investigation Record*, we find that the number recorded of cases of phthisis in husband and wife, within ten years, falls much short of the number that would probably have occurred in the practice of the observers supposing there to have been any infection at all in operation.

3. In most of the cases given in the *Record*, the persons supposed to have received direct infection lived under similar conditions, and for the most part in the same houses, and these conditions are often noted as having been very unhealthy. The infection is just as likely to have been indirect as direct, *i.e.*, from person to person.

4. If phthisis is directly contagious, it is remarkable that it should chiefly be contagious on certain soils ; and, further, it is difficult to see why drainage of the land should affect its contagiousness.

I have nowhere found any satisfactory proof of direct infection in a well-ventilated house, or even in the well-ventilated wards of a consumptive hospital, and this in spite of close contact, as in the attendance of a wife upon her husband, or in the nursing and sleeping together of near relatives and friends ; such an immunity, then, cannot be due merely to the disinfecting action of fresh air.

I may mention incidentally a striking example of the influence of soil which I investigated during the past year. The committee of the Hospital for Consumption, with which I am connected, had occasion to seek for a site for new wards. I had been struck with the freedom from the disease enjoyed by a portion of the locality in which I myself live, and it occurred to me that I might ascertain how many cases originated in the different parts of the district. A great portion of it is composed of deep, porous soil, but it is surrounded by boulder-clay, the result of glacial drift ; and a great part of Bowdon, and parts of Dunham and Altrincham, are built upon a thick bed of sand, in many places over 100 feet in thickness. The climate is thus rendered more temperate, and the air and soil drier.

After the wettest weather the paths speedily become dry, and the basement story of a house is often as dry as its attic. It has the further advantage that it is virgin soil. The sand is as pure and free from organic matter as in the days when it was deposited by ice-floes, or was silted up by the estuary of the Mersey. No house is ever built upon freshly-made ground, or on pits that have been filled up with refuse. The locality is well sewered, and has a plentiful supply of good water. Moreover, the inhabitants are for the most part well-to-do people. Out of 2,559 of population at the last census, only about 500 are poor, and live on the low-lying clay lands that surround the sandy downs upon which Bowdon is built. The remainder dwell in well-built, salubrious houses ; they are well fed, and comfortable in their circumstances.

It will thus be seen that such a community are in a position peculiarly well-fitted to preserve them from attacks of tubercular disease. I was, however, hardly prepared for the result of my inquiries.

Through the intervention of Sir W. Farr, I obtained from the superintendent registrar of deaths an extract from the death-register of all the deaths from diseases of the lungs occurring in Bowdon, in the ten years 1875–84. Of these, twenty-two were from phthisis, but eleven of them took place in the low-lying clay lands before mentioned, and nine of the remainder were found to have contracted the disease before coming to Bowdon. This leaves two to be accounted for, and one of these was a gentleman connected with the City Mission in Manchester, who was, therefore constantly obliged to attend crowded evening meetings in different parts of the town. The other was a merchant's clerk, who went to town at eight every morning, and did not return until seven p.m.

No woman or child died of the complaint ; in other words, the disease did not originate in any of the stationary population, resident during the ten years upon the sandy portion of the district.

It is certainly difficult to see why the condition of the soil should so greatly affect the distribution of the disease if it is mainly propagated by direct infection.

Another argument, which I owe to my friend Dr W. H. Broadbent (the late Sir W. H. B.), may be found in the frequency of cases of one-sided phthisis.

It is on these grounds that I venture to affirm the doubtfulness, or at least the extreme rarity, of direct contagion in phthisis. The very cases that are claimed by the contagionists as evidence of direct infection may therefore often be taken as proof of the existence of infected areas ; and thus I think that I am justified, in support of my theory, in calling attention to any instance in which phthisis has prevailed especially in certain localities, in certain streets, and even in certain houses.

My own attention was first called to the subject by some cases occurring in my own neighbourhood. One striking instance was that of a whole family of six members carried off by the disease in one house, the mother, an old woman, alone surviving. In another family, again, four or five children were thus disposed of, one of them, a son, dying in another house after he had contracted the disease at home ; but a daughter who was in service escaped altogether. In two other instances several members of each family died of the disease within short periods of one another.

The important feature of all these cases was that they occurred in small, badly ventilated cottages situated upon clay soils. The *Collective Investigation Record* contains a number of similar observations.

Dr Bampton, of Plymouth (No. 193), supplies three such instances, in one of which a family, consisting of a mother and nine children, all died of phthisis, the father remaining healthy ; several of the grandchildren also died of tubercular diseases, and not in the same house.

Nos. 159, 165, 168, 178, and 188 are also very striking cases. In most of these instances it is expressly mentioned that the houses in which the patients lived were small and ill-ventilated.

One observer, Dr J. S. Dewar, of Arbroath, remarks that in all his cases (No. 166) "the patients lived in small, confined houses, and slept in the 'box-beds' in use in Scotland." "During twenty-five years," he says, "I have not seen one case of contagion in the airy houses of the well-to-do."

I think one may reasonably doubt, therefore, whether the contagion was not indirect, and due mainly to the intensifying power of the atmospheric impurities. In two or three instances the virus certainly seems to have been introduced from without into houses previously entirely free from the disease.

Thus : No. 188. I. McI., aged 21, student, son of healthy parents, both living, no family history of phthisis ; took ill with a cough while studying in Glasgow in 1870, neglected it, came home at the end of the session, cough got worse, found both lungs tuberculous, died of phthisis in nine months. Had one sister, 19, and one brother, 17. The former a perfectly healthy girl, nursed her brother closely, got ill shortly after his death, and was dead in five months after him of phthisis. The brother, who slept with I. McI. during part of his illness, and wore his clothes after his death, showed symptoms of failing health before the sister died, and in about eighteen months died of phthisis. Parents still living in 1883.

No. 194. In 1862 a servant came home to her mother (a widow with three sons and two daughters, all grown up, father dead of epithelioma) suffering from phthisis. The house, consisting of two rooms and an attic, and lying under the brow of a hill on its northern aspect, was ill-ventilated and worse lighted. By the end of 1868 the only survivor of this family was a thin, delicate girl, who took little or no part in the nursing. They all died of phthisis, the mother dying last, between fifty and sixty years old.

No. 196.   A young man of the Indian navy came home suffering from phthisis. In a few months two of his sisters were taken with the same complaint, and died. A third sister married, and soon afterwards died of the same complaint; the young man also died. Later on the father was similarly affected, and died. After his death the widow became phthisical, and died also. Four years covered the whole outbreak, that is, from the arrival of this young man from India. The father was originally a very strong, healthy man, and all the children healthy up to about twenty or twenty-one, or even later. One sister still lives, and is now between forty and fifty.

No. 255 is a somewhat similar case.

The London Medical Record for July, 1884, quotes a case by Dr Kempf, of Louisville, tending towards the same conclusion, namely, that the disease may be introduced into a dwelling from without, and also that it may be eradicated from it. I do not think it proves anything more, for I should greatly doubt the statement that the convent in question was well ventilated. The story is, however, as follows :

In 1880 the Sisters' Convent, in the village of Ferdinand, was entirely free from consumption ; it is well ventilated, is high and dry, and is well drained. In the autumn of 1880, a girl of 18 was found to be consumptive. She continued to sleep in the general dormitory. One sister after another now commenced with similar symptoms, and in four months after the first case began there were nine cases in sisters who had been thought to be exceptionally healthy. Four sisters died in the course of a year. After complete isolation of the sick, the epidemic was stopped.

These cases in themselves would be sufficient to show the probability that phthisis may become, at any rate for a time, epidemic in certain houses.

It seemed to be probable also that a research into the intimate history of some of the unhealthy districts of our large towns would supply similar evidence, and I have therefore undertaken an inquiry into the distribution of phthisis in certain parts of Manchester and Salford. In this inquiry I have been much assisted by the admirable manner in which the records of mortality are kept in both these towns, and the mode in which they are broken up, for statistical and other purposes, into small and manageable areas.

I have also to thank the officials of the health offices of the respective corporations of these towns, and especially Mr Dawson, of Manchester, and Dr Tatham, Medical Officer of Salford, for the readiness with which they came to my assistance, and for the excellent mortality tables that they had prepared for me of the districts in question.

In Manchester, almost at haphazard, I selected a small part of Ancoats, of which a map is here given.

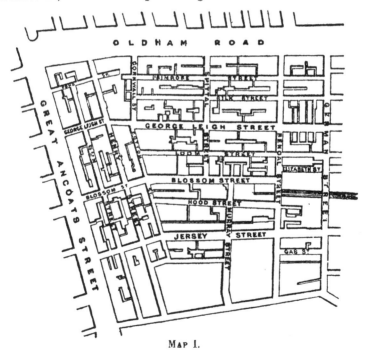

MAP 1.

The following description of this district is given by Mr Leigh, Medical Officer of Health, in his *Report*, published in 1884 :

"Nearly the whole of the houses in the district were built before the year 1830.   There are a great number of back-to-back houses in all parts of the district.   The width of the streets ranges from 30 feet to 4 feet, the greater number of them being 16 feet or 17 feet wide.   The passages vary in width, and are only 2 feet 6 inches wide in some instances ; in many cases the backs of the houses are too near to each other.

"The streets are for the most part paved and sewered.   The houses, as a rule, are without cellars, and have no ventilating spaces under the floors.   They rise directly from the ground ; the outside walls are 9 inches thick, and the inside walls are $4\frac{1}{2}$ inches or 3 inches thick.   They smell fusty ; the ceilings of some are only 6 feet from the floor ; the timber of many is in a state of decay.   Houses in such a condition, and so erected, cannot be otherwise than damp.   The absence of any provision to prevent the moisture of the ground rising into the walls, and the thinness of the latter affording so little defence against rain, the interior can seldom or never be as dry as a house should be.   From the want of subjacent ventilation any emanation from the soil must find immediate vent into the houses."   The population is about 5,600 persons.

The first thing that strikes one in looking through the mortality tables is the large number of deaths from tubercular disease— 150 in five years in a population of 5,600—thirty each year—5·3 per 1,000.

2.   Although these deaths are scattered about throughout the district, about 15 per cent. take place in the narrow courts opening by passages into the streets.

3.   The longest and widest streets are Jersey Street, with ten deaths, and George Leigh Street, with eight ; but the number of deaths in these streets is approached by the mortality of eight in Hood Street, half their length—a short lane blocked at each end— Silk Street and Primrose Street, each with nine deaths.   Henry Street, a long thoroughfare, has only four deaths, whilst Bond Street, a *cul-de-sac* one quarter its length, has seven.

4.   The coincidences of deaths from phthisis in the same house

within the space of five years are also most common in the more confined areas.

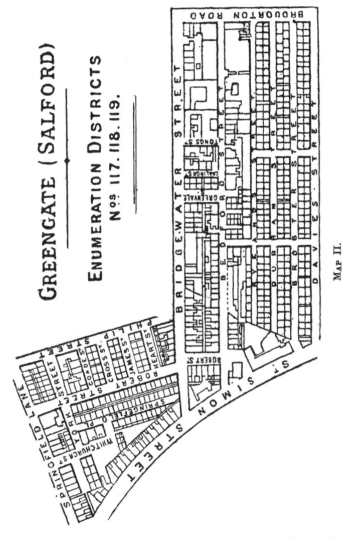

MAP II.

Thus there are two deaths in the same house at No. 2, Chapel Court, three at No. 13, Bond Street, and two at No. 18. There are three deaths at No. 10, Jepson's Court, and two at No. 3.

Two at No. 3, Hewitt's Court ; and in Hood Street there are two deaths each at three houses, Nos. 2, 36 and 45.   In Spittal Street there are two such coincidences, one at No. 12, and another at No. 29.   In Gun Street there are two deaths at No. 43 ; in Blossom Street two at No. 52 ; and in Berwick's Court there are three at No. 5.   In Lorne Street there are two at No. 2.   In the rest of the district there are, in Henry Street, four cases of such coincidences, at Nos. 9, 20, 30 and 52 ; in Bengal Street one at No. 31 ; and in Jersey Street one at No. 29.

ENUMERATION DISTRICT N? 3.

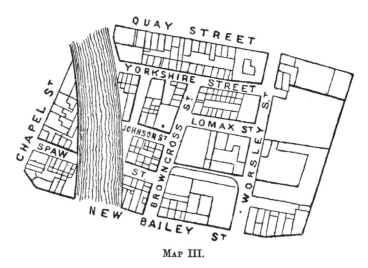

MAP III.

Altogether there are twenty-one such coincidences, or forty-four deaths, and fifteen of them (thirty in all) occur in the narrow streets, *culs-de-sac*, or small courts.

In Salford the districts into which it is divided are much smaller than those in Manchester, in fact they are the enumeration districts adopted at the last census ; but Dr Tatham, the Medical Officer of Health, kindly selected three contiguous portions, with a total population of 2,609, and he gave me the particulars of their mortality, taken for the six years 1879–85, and had the accompanying map drawn for me (see Map II).

Dr Tatham also provided me with similar materials for another district—No. 3, Regent Road; and he personally visited the Greengate districts with me, and verified the causes of death recorded. I am greatly indebted to him for the kind interest that he took in my inquiry, and for the great assistance that he afforded to me.

It will be seen from the map that these districts are simpler in their construction than the Ancoats district. There are fewer courts and alleys, but the streets are almost wholly composed of back-to-back houses ; and whilst some of them are thoroughfares, others, notably Durham Street and Rylands Street, and Springfield Terrace or Place, are closed at one end. This construction enables us to compare the streets more readily, and we shall find that their respective phthisis-rates bear out the conclusions at which we have arrived with respect to Ancoats.

In Greengate district, No. 117 (Map II), with 892 inhabitants, there are in the six years forty-seven deaths from tubercular disease, and of these twenty took place in Durham Street, which is blocked at one end, and nine in Rylands Street (on one side only), all in the single or back-to-back houses, and thirteen of these are in groups of two or more in the same house. In Broster Street, also entirely composed of back-to-back houses, and with its ventilation checked by a curve at the end nearest St Simon Street, there are thirteen tubercular deaths, two of them at the same house, No. 66.

On the other side of Rylands Street, in No. 118 district, there were only two such deaths, and it is interesting to note, that although the cottages are just as small as the others, they have an outlet to the back.

In Bedford Street also, a broader street, mostly composed of similar cottages, opening at the back, there were only twelve tubercular deaths, and six of these were in the three houses Nos. 4, 11 and 41, in the worst part of the street ; and in the whole of this No. 118 district, with 880 inhabitants, there were only twenty-nine such deaths.

In No. 119 district, with 837 inhabitants, there are in all twenty-one tubercular deaths, and seven of these are in the short, narrow *cul-de-sac* called Springfield Terrace, two of them in one house, No. 9, whilst there is only one in the broad Robert Street, and one in Philip Street, and none in York Street.

These facts show that there, as in Ancoats, the streets most infected with phthisis are also the most confined and ill-ventilated, and that the larger proportion of deaths take place in the cave-like back-to-back dwellings.

Dr Tatham writes, with regard to the subsoil: "I have gathered from the surveyor, who has for years past been engaged in repairing the drains in this locality, that the subsoil underlying these districts is mainly clayey and alluvial. There is no accurate geological chart of the district."

In the Regent Road District, No. 3 (Map III), numbering 791 inhabitants, there were in the six years forty deaths from undoubted tubercular disease, which is as high an average as that of Greengate, but the arrangement of the houses is less regular, and there are many works interspersed amongst them. It is thus more difficult to make a comparison between the different parts of the district. There are also fewer back-to-back houses. Still, ten out of the forty cases occurred in five houses, *i.e.*, there were five coincidences of the disease in the same house, two of them in Quay Street, one in Shaw Street, one in Yorkshire Street, and one in a small court, Bennett's Square.

I am aware that there are certain sources of fallacy in drawing conclusions from these statistics. There is the possibility of wrong diagnosis, and, still more likely, there is the uncertainty as to whether the disease originated in the house in which the several deaths took place. In a working-class population, such as that in these districts, there are frequent changes of residence, and hence we cannot be sure that the same family has occupied the same house for any length of time.

I would point out, however, that errors in diagnosis may have been made in more than one direction, and that it is even more likely that a case of phthisis has passed undiscovered under the guise of bronchitis or pneumonia, than that the opposite mistake has been made.

The change of residence would also tell just as much against the view that I have taken of the results as in its favour, and, therefore, we may perhaps be allowed to set off one against the other.

There is yet another possibility, namely, that these poor sufferers might have drifted in their poverty from healthier houses into the cheap and unhealthy quarters in which they died. As a matter of fact, however, these work-people seldom leave the same district, though they may change their houses, and, as may be seen from the maps, the characteristics of the houses themselves are very much the same as regards accommodation, and their weekly rental varies very little in different streets.

On the whole I am inclined to accept the mortality tables as giving, if not an exact, yet a very fair, picture of the incidence of tubercular disease in the several parts of each district ; and I venture to think, that if the areas which we have found so much infested with tubercle were opened out and improved, we should find a great diminution in the amount of this disease ; and I claim them as, on the whole, supporting my hypothesis of the existence of specially infective areas, in which either polluted ground air or an atmosphere reeking with organic matter has given virulence to the organised germ of the disease, much in the same way as sewage, or polluted water, contribute to the conveyance of cholera and typhoid fever. And there is nothing in the natural history of tubercle that need run counter to this theory. Tubercle has been compared by Villemin to the granulations of glanders, and to the gummata of syphilis, and other observers have found analogies to it in the ulceration of Peyer's glands in enteric fever. It has further been shown, by Thiersch and Prof. Burdon Sanderson, that the virulence of the poison of cholera and typhoid fever increases after its extrusion from the body. There is, therefore, nothing unlikely in the hypothesis that contact with a certain kind of organic matter will assist the sporulation of the bacillus of tubercle, and render it more infective after a time than at the moment of its departure from the lungs of a phthisical patient.

It is on these grounds that I venture to propose my explanation of the mode in which tubercular diseases cling especially to certain localities, and to account for their spreading infectively in certain areas, whilst they are so rarely directly infectious from person to person.

(2) TUBERCULOSIS AND LEPROSY : A PARALLEL AND A PROPHECY[1]

THE LANCET, *July* 11, 1896

TUBERCLE is the twin-sister of leprosy. The likeness between the two diseases is remarkable, and the points of resemblance are so numerous that we are encouraged to draw a parallel between them. It is possible, indeed, not only to compare them together, but also to draw conclusions from the past history of one of them, leprosy, which may shed light upon the probable course in the near future of the other, tuberculosis. In other words, from a consideration of the circumstances attending the decline of leprosy we may venture to make a forecast as to the probable date of the final disappearance of tuberculosis from our midst. Let us first trace their close relationship : (1) in their specific causation and in their morphology ; (2) in their pathology ; (3) in their distribution ; (4) in their general history and the conditions favourable or otherwise to their existence ; and (5) in their infectiveness and hereditary transmission.

1. *Their etiology and morphology.* Each affection is characterised by the presence of a bacillus, and, although the lepra bacillus is sometimes slightly clubbed at one end, the two microbes are so similar that they can often scarcely be distinguished, either microscopically or by means of the tests applied to them. They take the same stains, though at slightly different rates, and the lepra bacillus is less easily decolourised by certain reagents than that of tubercle. It is also grouped within the lepra cells more thickly than the tubercle bacillus is usually distributed. It is hardly, if at all, inoculable, and cannot readily be cultivated like tubercle. These are, however, comparatively trifling distinctions. The most important difference between them lies in their respective points of attack. The bacillus of leprosy chiefly affects the skin and mucous membranes, the nerves, and the bones ; tubercle the ungs, the lymphatic glands, and the serous membranes. Yet they

---

[1] A paper read before the Epidemiological Society, May 15, 1896.

are both able to attack almost every part of the body. The bacillus of tubercle often seizes upon the bones, and has been found in the nervous tissues, whilst that of leprosy is not unfrequently discovered in the lungs. On the whole, it is perhaps not surprising that some physicians, amongst whom we must place Dr Daniellsen, the great authority on leprosy, are inclined to believe from a study of their morphology that the diseases are identical in character and that their bacilli are modifications of one species altered only by their environment.

2. *Their pathology.* The similarity which we have observed in the micro-organisms of these diseases is carried forward in their pathological action. The structure both of tubercle and the lepra knots shows that they are alike produced by slow inflammatory action, due to the specific irritation of their respective organisms. They both travel infectively through the body, spreading chiefly along the track of the lymphatics ; both usually have periods of latency or quiescence of longer or shorter duration ; and both are capable of natural cure, *i.e.* by the unaided powers of nature ; but they both tend to a fatal issue. The main point of difference in this regard between the two diseases is the greater chronicity of leprosy, which lasts on the average ten or twelve years, instead of three or four, which is now the ordinary duration of tubercle.

3. *Their distribution.* Both are distinctly "endemic" diseases, remaining for long periods in the same districts, varying little, if at all, in their rate of progress, independent of climate and season ; but both are aggravated by overcrowding of dwellings, by dampness of subsoil, and by filthy surroundings. Leprosy, like tubercle, affects all classes of society, though both are more common amongst the poor and filthy· than amongst the rich and cleanly. They both appear amongst the well-fed as well as amongst those who are half-starved ; and, though certain races of mankind are more prone to these diseases than others, none are entirely exempt if other conditions are favourable. The proofs of some of these statements are to be found in a study of Leloir's map of the distribution of leprosy throughout the world and in a comparison between it and Lombard's map of the distribution of tubercle. In their localisation these complaints closely resemble one another, except that at the present day leprosy is absent from the British

Isles and from the greater part of Europe, whilst tubercle is therein widely spread. On the other hand, leprosy is much more common than tubercle in Siberia, in Iceland, and generally in the islands of the world. But when we consider the ancient spread of leprosy, as well as that of to-day, it becomes evident that the phrase " a ubiquitous disease " is as applicable to leprosy as it is to tubercle. The other assertions made are also confirmed by the history of the diseases in every place that they have attacked[1]. The parallel only fails when we come to compare :

4. *The peculiar conditions under which each disease is able to exist and spread infectively.* That these conditions are not exactly the same is evident, otherwise the same causes that have contributed to the decline, and ultimately to the extinction, of leprosy in most of the countries of Europe would equally have prevailed against tubercle. This, as we are only too well aware, is not the case, seeing that the latter disease is still much more widely spread amongst us than leprosy ever was.

As we have already seen, there is now no question as to the specific causes of these affections. They are both bacillary diseases ; and as such the organisms, in order to produce the complaints, must be communicable, whether by contact, by inoculation, by fœtal transmission, or by air, food, or drink ; but every person is not necessarily seized after exposure to these sources of infection ; in each disease the body can only become infected under certain conditions ; and it is these all-important conditions, and their connecting links, that must now be studied. It is probably the

---

[1] Dr Thin says (*Leprosy*, p. 185) : " There is a close analogy between the two parasites. They both may gain admission into the human frame without leaving any trace at the point of entrance ; they both have an uncertain period of incubation ; they both may develop rapidly or very slowly ; and in both instances, once admission and development have taken place, the complete extinction of the parasite, if it ever does so, occurs with extreme rarity ; although in both cases the parasite may be limited to certain isolated parts of the body and may live very quiescent over a long period of years, the death of the patient in process of time probably taking place from some other disease. Of the two parasites, the tubercle bacillus develops the strongest poison, and thus can mercifully kill the victim without producing extraordinary ravages and mutilations like those that take place before the patient succumbs to the enormous development of the leprosy bacillus which is compatible with life."

neglect of this study in the past, that has led to much of the controversy that has been carried on with regard to their communicability. In this research perhaps we may find some features that
are common to both diseases, and others that may serve to account
for the differences in their distribution in time and locality. It
will be necessary, then, to examine somewhat closely the nature
of the predisposing causes of the two diseases, and at the outset I
would point out that these conditions may properly be grouped
under two chief headings : (A) the bodily conditions predisposing
to each disease ; and (B) the conditions of environment that tend
to keep alive, or to increase the virulence of, the respective organisms of leprosy and tuberculosis.

(A) It is not needful to say much under the first head with
regard to tubercle. The causes of bodily predisposition to this
disease have been thoroughly investigated and only require
enumeration to be at once recognised. They are : (*a*) hereditary
weakness of organs or of constitution rendering the body vulnerable by the bacillus ; (*b*) susceptibility to the disease acquired by
habits of life, occupations, etc. ; (*c*) the influence of age, sex, and
race ; (*d*) the predisposing influence of previous diseases—either
general diseases of the system or local injuries and disorders of the
lungs themselves ; and (*e*) a diet lacking in fatty matter. But
when we come to consider the causes that increase the receptivity
of the body to leprosy we have a somewhat more difficult task.
It is, indeed, generally supposed that abrasions and wounds of the
surface are necessary to the reception of the virus, mainly because
exposed parts, such as the hands, feet, and face, are most commonly
the places where the disease commences, and because of the
acknowledged difficulty of producing infection by contact or even
by inoculation ; but this circumstance would not account for the
dying out of the complaint in Central Europe, for we cannot suppose
that such injuries became less common in more recent times.
Again, some authorities believe that hereditary tendencies count
for much in the susceptibility to leprosy. Amongst these we may
cite Dr Daniellsen, Dr Neisser, and Dr Zambuco. But, on the
other hand, Dr Hansen states that of 160 Norwegian lepers who
had settled in the States of Wisconsin, Minnesota, and Dakota
none of the offspring—in some cases as far as the great-great-

grandchildren—have shown signs of the disease. He points out
also that there could have been no question of heredity in the case
of the great outbreak of leprosy in Hawaii. In any case heredity
cannot have been of supreme importance, otherwise the disease
would not have declined as it has done. In order to find out the
essential conditions of its spread, the most hopeful course to pursue
is to compare the social state of the people in mediæval Europe
with that which prevailed at, or about, the time of its decline and
final disappearance ; and, to check our conclusions, we may note
to what extent the conditions we have marked are now to be
found in the places where the complaint is still prevalent and
advancing. This work has already been very thoroughly done
by several writers—most recently by Dr Newman in his prize
essay on the History of the Decline and Final Extinction of Leprosy
as an Endemic Disease in the British Isles (National Leprosy
Fund). In a very able fashion this writer passes in review all the
possible causes to which the susceptibility of populations may be
due—absence of sanitation, poverty, dampness of soil, overcrowding, hereditary taint, inoculation, etc.; but he dismisses them
all as not really active agents in its promotion. He finally selects
"dietetics" as the "only possible active cause left by the elimina-
tion and exclusion of the others." It may be remarked that in
this conclusion he is by no means alone ; he is supported, for
instance, by Mr Jonathan Hutchinson and by the reporters to the
first Commission of the Royal College of Physicians of London on
the subject; but it is right to mention that others, notably Dr Thin
and the second Commission of the same body, took a different
view and gave in their adhesion to the "contagion" theory. In
this contention, cases are brought forward to show that the disease
may be contracted when nothing wrong in the diet can be pointed
out, just as persons have been known to become tuberculous who
are well-fed in every respect. Yet in both diseases diet may be
one of the predisposing causes ; and it is hard to resist the strong
evidence that this is certainly the case with regard to leprosy.
Under the head of diet mere starvation is not included, for " poverty
of food, provided this be fresh and wholesome, is insufficient to
produce or perpetuate the disease[1]." Nor is it simply a " fish "

[1] Report of the Commission of the Royal College of Physicians of London, 1867.

diet ; any unnatural food will predispose to it, but especially salt and semi-putrid fish foods. On this point it may be well to make a few selections from the mass of evidence, drawn from many sources by Dr Newman, first, as to the diet of the people in the Middle Ages, and next, as to the change of custom in this respect just before and during the decline of the disease in Europe. Thus he quotes Larry, who ascribes the leprosy from which the French suffered in Egypt to the unwholesome character of the pork ; Forrestus and others, who believed that the leprosy of the Middle Ages in England was due to the salt, putrid, indigestible food that was eaten, and the frequent scarcity of that owing to the disorder of the times. Exactly the same view was promulgated by the Royal College of Physicians of London in 1867. They call attention to the " scarcity of fresh meat during the Middle Ages and the ordinary consumption of highly salted meats, the scanty supply of vegetables and fruits, and the inferior and often unsound character of the bread in common use." In St Kilda leprosy was ascribed " to gross feeding, and that on those fat fowls, the fulmar and solan geese, the latter of which they keep for a whole year without any salt or pepper to preserve them." Uncooked meat and other " gross aliments " are said to have caused leprosy in Ireland ; half-rotten flesh or fish in the Färöe Islands. These views are supported by historical evidence, collected from various sources, as to the diet and social condition of the people of England in these early times. Only one or two examples of these can be given. From the kitchen accounts of Humphrey, Duke of Buckinghamshire (1443 to 1444) we learn of the purchase and storage of " 10 barrels salt herrings, 11 cades fresh herrings, 6 cades sprats, 3379 salt fish, 3060 stock-fish, 6 barrels salt salmon, 1 barrel cod, 1 barrel and 13 salt eels, 1 barrel sturgeons, 12 lampreys, 1 pair of porpoises."

In 1446, at the feast to commemorate the instalment of George Nevile as Archbishop of York, 608 pikes and 12 porpoises were used. At a similar ceremony in 1504, when Warham was made Archbishop of Canterbury, the following quantity of fish was used : 300 ling, 600 cod, 7 barrels of salted salmon, 40 fresh salmon, 14 barrels of white herrings, 20 cades of red herrings (600 herrings in each cade), 5 barrels of salted sturgeons, 2 barrels of salted eels,

600 fresh eels, 8000 whelks, 500 pikes, 400 tenches, 100 carp, 800 bream, 2 barrels of salted lampreys, 1400 fresh lampreys, 134 salted congers, 200 great roaches, and a quantity of seals, porpoises, and other fish. This feast occurred, as it is stated, on a "fish day." It was said that "eels were used as abundantly as swine." Before the Reformation, indeed, "for nearly one hundred days in the year only fish could be used because of the numerous fasts, so salt fish must have gone practically all over populated England ; and it is quite certain that a good deal of storage went on." In the latter part of the fourteenth century, in the reign of Edward III, an Act was passed to regulate the traffic in salted fish ; it is evident, therefore, that before this period much fish had been dried, salted and secretly stored. It is probable that this Act in some measure diminished the consumption of this article of diet, and that with the rise of Protestantism a still greater change in this direction took place. It was about this time that leprosy began sensibly to decline in this country. This evidence will perhaps be sufficient as far as mediæval dietetics are concerned, and with the exception of China Dr Newman makes also a good case against the food in countries now afflicted by leprosy. With regard to China the only thing that he can find to say is that "much pork is used and quantities of *excellent* fish and shell-fish." In India "the ordinary diet of the natives is rice" with some herbs gathered out of the fields, but a good deal of fish is also eaten. "Dried fish is used all round the coast, especially in the Madras presidency and Burma. In the latter country dried fish, more or less in a state of decomposition, is almost universally eaten, but in small quantities." Reference is made to the report of the Royal College of Physicians of London, 1867, to show that a fish diet, inland or on the coast, is not a rare diet. Concerning Icelanders Vontroil says : "Their continual occupation is fishing ; they are night and day exposed to wet and cold, frequently fed upon corrupted rotten fish, fish livers and roe, fat and train of whale and sea-dogs, as likewise congealed and stale sour milk." "Nine-tenths of them know not the luxury of bread or vegetables" (Henderson). In New Zealand the natives lived on very restricted supplies of food. They had no quadrupeds and but few edible vegetables. They lived near the seashore and very largely on what

the sea produced. " As regards the Englishmen who became lepers (very few indeed), it is thought probable that they got it from eating the same food as the Maories and not from contagion. It did not spread in their families nor did their children inherit it.... Dr Myles[1] states that even so far back as the time of Captain Cook leprosy prevailed in New Zealand, but only on the shores of an inland lake where fish diet was used and nowhere else." In Japan " the diet of the people, especially the lower orders, largely consists of fish, often raw." With reference to a recent increase of leprosy in the Sandwich Islands Dr Arning is quoted as saying " that although the use of fish as food had always been common it was only quite recently that it had been salted. Probably it was this recent use of salted fish which had caused the outbreak." Dr Donnet attributes leprosy in Portugal to Newfoundland salted fish. Dr Hjort says the same of the Färöe Islands. Speaking of leprosy at the Cape, Dr Wright says : " Anything that tends to lower the system would render the subject more liable to take the disease. It is due more to overcrowded dwellings in which people live like pigs. I think that, not the fish diet, but the decomposing fish around them is the more probable cause. Decomposing fish is more injurious than any other decaying matter."

It is upon these grounds that Dr Newman bases his advocacy of the " diet " doctrine ; and we may grant that he has strong reasons for believing that a certain diet does predispose to the disease. If this be so, then we have the further likeness between leprosy and tubercle that bodily predisposition is an important factor in the spread of each disease, though the causes of the susceptibility may be different in the two cases. The necessity for such predisposition is perhaps less in tubercle than in leprosy, for there can be no doubt that, when the surrounding conditions are sufficiently bad, the former disease can attack the healthiest individuals, and those who have no hereditary tendency to it. But it will be obvious also that the chief bodily predisposing influence in the case of leprosy has not the same effect upon tubercle. The rank fish foods have no determining effect upon the latter disease, but absence of fatty matter in the diet probably has. It is, perhaps, owing to these distinctive differences that

[1] Royal Academy of Medicine in Ireland.

phthisis is conspicuous by its absence in several parts of the world where leprosy is still rampant, as in Siberia, Iceland, the Färöe Islands, and St Kilda ; but it is yet only too common in places from which leprosy has entirely disappeared.

(B) Next, as to the conditions of environment that tend to keep alive, or to increase the virulence of, the respective organisms of leprosy and tuberculosis. First, with regard to leprosy, it is probable that Dr Newman goes too far when he affirms " that it may be taken for granted that contagion is not a chief cause of the propagation of leprosy in modern times." At any rate, the other writers of prize essays, Dr Ehlers and Dr Impey, and also Dr Thin, differ entirely from him on this point. Dr Thin shows (p. 137) that "leprosy when it has spread has always done so in continuity with previously existing foci." We can, therefore, only concede to Dr Newman that not merely the infecting germ is needed but also a susceptible state of the body, and that the predisposition is most commonly produced by unwholesome food. The infecting germ also needs a medium in which it can live. It is quite true that the lepra bacillus is very difficult to cultivate outside the body ; but history and analogy both lead us to believe that it can retain its virulence in a filthy environment much longer than it can in cleanly houses. Dr Newman's own historical survey contains ample proof that the conditions surrounding the populations attacked by leprosy were, and are, such as would tend to assist contagion.

It is not necessary to go deeply into the proofs of this assertion ; it will be sufficient to quote a few passages bearing upon the point. " In all the towns of Europe the streets were unpaved and ill-constructed ; every sort of filth was permitted to be thrown into the streets and remain there ; vaults and common sewers were seldom adopted and the drains ran above ground ; the office and duty of scavenger was imperfectly executed or neglected ; the supply of water was deficient, and the narrowness of the streets prevented any free circulation of air." " From the thirteenth to the sixteenth century most of the towns of England and Europe were in the condition above described. The streets of London were filled with common lay-stalls of all manner of filth and garbage, which the people were in vain ordered to remove from their own doors ; the sewers, the few that existed, were much more harm than good, and large drains ran above ground ; the access of air into the narrow streets was prevented by the projecting houses, which almost met at the top, and the intervening space below was filled up with enormous sign boards." Erasmus, in his often quoted letter to Cardinal Wolsey, says : " The homes of the people were wooden or mud houses, small and dirty, without drainage or ventilation ; the floors, of earth or clay, were covered with rushes, straw, and other rubbish, which were occasionally renewed, but underneath lay unmolested an ancient collection of beer, grease, fragments of fish, spittle, the excrements of dogs and cats, and everything that is nasty." Close by the doors stood " the mixen," a collection of every abomination, streams of filth from which polluted the houses and neighbourhood, including any river at hand. " Soap was scarcely used at all, and certainly to the labourer was a luxury he could rarely afford to buy, hence a life of dirt in consequence. He slept upon heaps of decayed vegetable refuse, and yet there were no fresh vegetables to eat." The clothing was chiefly of wool, and was rarely changed. " The use of linen changes, shirts or shifts, in the room of sordid and filthy woollen long worn next the skin, is a matter of neatness and comparatively modern," and so on. Similar accounts are given of the peoples of China, India, and Iceland at the present day, and attention is called to the un-drained, damp condition of the soil.

Dr Ehlers believes that leprosy in Iceland is entirely due to the environment, and he gives the following graphic description of the " badstofa," the Icelander's dwelling. " If you enter this badstofa when thirteen or fourteen persons lie sleeping there, first of all you feel a temperature which certainly, both summer and winter, reminds you of the tepidarium of a Roman bath, but surely here the likeness ceases. A suffocating stink and an unwholesome smell meet you. It is the smell of the mouldy hay, of the sheep-skin quilts that are never dried or aired ; it is the smell of the dirt which is dragged into the house on the clumsy Icelandic skin shoes that want double soles, and are quite unqualified to keep out the dampness. In this dirt a confused mixture of cats, dogs, and children lie reeking on the floor exchanging caresses and echino-cocci ; it is the smell of the wet stockings and the woollen shirts.

which hang to dry next to a slice of dried halibut ('Reckling') or the dried cod's head, this dreadful irrational favourite dish, for which the Icelander pays four kroner [4s. 6d.] a hundred. And if you poke your nose into the corner of the badstofa you will find a bucket in which the urine of the whole party is gathered; it is considered good for wool-washing. One must have seen and smelt it all to be able to understand that the leprous disease is due neither to the rancid butter nor to the dry fish. Just as well as raising accusations against these articles of food which certain leprologists do, one might complain of the want of brooms to sweep the floor with, or insist that the leprosy is owing to the want of window-hooks or to the stagnant water that they drink. It is neither the one nor the other of these factors, but the whole ensemble; it is the absolute want of cleanliness plus Armauer Hansen's bacillus which in such an interior finds its true paradise. The rancid oil or butter is only a symptom of the general filthiness which manures the soil in which the disease thrives." Dr Ehlers speaks scornfully of the "fish-diet" theory, of the idea that the introduction of the potato has led to a diminution of the disease, for as he says : " At the present time the potato has found its way to most of the Icelanders' tables, but unfortunately the leprous disease is on the increase." " Is now this," he says, " maybe, the potato's fault ? " Like Dr Newman, he considers that " this disease can strike root there where Hansen's bacillus re-finds its favourite soil of uncleanliness, bad nourishment, and filthiness, under hygienic circumstances which have not altered in many respects since the Middle Ages."

Whether or not the poison of leprosy is directly introduced into the body in unwholesome food, which seems very unlikely, or is communicated from without through the skin, the external conditions that have just been described are only too well adapted to keep alive the virus, and to facilitate its entrance into a suscep- tible person. In several points, as we have already seen, the con- ditions favourable to leprosy touch those that help forward tubercle, notably the overcrowding, and the want of proper drainage of the subsoil of dwellings; but, as we have already seen with respect to diet, so also the surrounding conditions that assist, or rather that are essential to the one disease, cannot be identical with those that are mainly instrumental in bringing about the other. The filth of Siberia, Iceland, and St Kilda has not been able to propagate the virus of tubercle as well as that of leprosy. Apparently, also, although laboratory experiments do not demonstrate the fact, the distribution of the two diseases tends to show that the lepra bacillus stands cold better than that of tubercle. The specific influence favourable to the spread of tubercle is undoubtedly " foul air " polluted with organic matter from an impure subsoil, or, still more potent for evil, air polluted by emanations from the lungs and bodies of human beings crowded together within small areas, organic products scarcely diluted by the scanty supplies of outer air that make their way into the close dwelling-rooms, and seldom swept away by true ventilation. It is unnecessary to accumulate proofs of this now well-recognised fact, but we may again recall the terrible experience of the British army before 1855 in all parts of the world, the history of overcrowded public institutions, and the tubercle-infected areas of our large towns. The contrast, also, between the incidence of the disease upon populations living an open-air life, and upon those aggregated together in ill-drained, badly-ventilated, closely-packed tenements, is sufficient to indicate the true source of the evil. When leprosy died out of Mid-Europe it is probable that in the above-mentioned respects the people were no better off, if not worse, than they were before, and hence, although this disease slowly dwindled away, tubercle was as rampant as ever.

Lastly (5), we have to consider yet another singular resemblance between tubercle and leprosy—namely, the curious coincidence that the questions of their transmission by contagion, and by hereditary descent, are still hotly disputed amongst the physicians of our time, especially amongst those who are likely to be best acquainted with these disorders. I need only cite Dr Hansen and Dr Daniellsen of Norway, who are on opposite sides, with reference to the contagion and the hereditary nature of leprosy, and Dr Baumgarten and Dr Bollinger in regard to tubercle. It is true that these disputes are only matters of opinion ; but underlying them, and causing the difference of opinion, there are fundamental points of resemblance. In both, the difficulty of proving contagion arises from the length of time that may elapse between the reception of the virus and the outbreak of the disease ; in both, there is the necessity for some anterior existence, or preparation, of a fertile bodily soil upon which the organism can germinate ; and in both, there is the abundance of infecting material everywhere spread abroad. Again, in regard to the question of inheritance, there is interposed, in the case of each disease, the stumbling block that the surroundings of families are usually similar, rendering it difficult to say whether the disease was favoured by hereditary weakness or by the environment. Looking back, then, for a moment, we have seen that these disorders are alike (1) in their etiology, (2) in their pathology, (3) in their course and distribution, and (4) in many points in their natural history. We can, therefore, say that they run upon closely parallel lines ; but that, in spite of their remarkable similarity, they cannot be regarded as absolutely identical, as they are still by some authorities ; nor can we accept Mr Hutchinson's opinion that the differences between them may possibly be only acquired and temporary[1]. Notwithstanding the differences that we have marked between the two diseases, however, I venture to think that they are at least so far alike, as to make it permissible, from a study of the decline of one complaint, and its causes, to attempt to glean some idea of the most hopeful means of diminishing the other ; and that we may even go on further and prophesy that, as one disease, leprosy, has disappeared from our midst, so the other, tubercle, may also be made to vanish, and that from the recognition of its predisposing causes we may learn in what way it may best be attacked, and finally driven from amongst civilised nations.

1.   The first lesson to be learnt from a review of the history of the disease is the fact that leprosy was banished mainly by general sanitary measures, by reforms in the modes of feeding, by better clothing, and probably to some extent by greater cleanliness of houses and persons.

2.   That it was scarcely affected by direct efforts at preventing contagion.   All the authorities are agreed that segregation of the lepers in lazar houses had little or nothing to do with its decline. Dr Newman shows " that strict segregation never was carried out in England."   Dr Ehlers declares that the four hospitals founded

---

[1] *Brit. Med. Journ.* March 8th, 1890.

in Iceland in 1651 "never got to contain many of the leprous
patients, hardly more than 5 per cent. of the whole number."
The Chief Rabbi of the Jews, the Rev. Dr Adler, writes to Dr Thin :
" The uncleanness of the leper seems, according to the Talmud, to
have been an ordinance for the purpose of securing Levitical purity,
and not for the purpose of preventing contagion. For this reason
the heathen or stranger when a leper was not considered unclean."
Dr Thin himself, though an advocate for isolation, yet remarks :
" It is evident that the vitality of the bacillus lepræ, which has
kept the organism alive in successive generations for four or five
thousands of years (and who can tell how much longer ?), is
nevertheless associated with conditions that render its transmission
from one host to another an operation which is only successful
by a combination of circumstances that, fortunately for the
human race, take place comparatively exceptionally." In other
words, if the conditions favourable to its spread are done away
with, the decline of the disease is certain, and it need not be a
terror to mankind. Much the same may be said of tubercle.
Segregation is still less necessary for the prevention of this disease
than for that of leprosy. No attempt at isolation has hitherto
been made in this country for the suppression of phthisis ; and yet,
as we shall see presently, the disease is gradually disappearing.
In the next place, applying what we have learned with regard to
leprosy, we may fairly expect that tubercle will be amenable, first,
to general sanitary measures, and second, to care in regard to diet.
It is, indeed, probable that tubercle can more easily be stamped
out than leprosy, and it is likely that if the work is once fairly
undertaken it will be more successful than a crusade against leprosy.
The bacillus of tubercle, though very tenacious of life under certain
conditions, is in truth a very tender plant. (1) In the form of
tuberculous dust it is destroyed by a short exposure to direct sunlight, or even diffuse daylight. Free currents of fresh air, also,
soon diminish its virulence or destroy its power. We can affirm
these facts, not only as a deduction from the history of the disease,
but also by an appeal to direct experiment. In a research carried
out in 1889 by Professor Dreschfeld and myself[1] it was found that

---

[1] *Proceedings of the Royal Society*, vol. XLIX. p. 66. (See also p. 142 of this volume.)

sputum, exposed to the air in a poor, badly-drained cottage, retained its virulence for two or three months at least; but the same material, freely exposed to air and light in a hospital for phthisis, and in a well-lighted, well-ventilated, and well-drained house, entirely lost its power of communicating the disease even by inoculation into rabbits. More recently Professor Delépine joined me in the work, and we made an attempt to determine how short a period of exposure to air and light would suffice to destroy the virulent action of the microbe[1]. The minimum time of exposure to air alone, *i.e.* in the dark, was not fully ascertained, for after three days of such exposure tubercle was produced, though it was evident that the power of the virus was already somewhat attenuated. On the other hand, all the specimens exposed to both air and light, even for two days only and for one hour of sunshine, were found to have entirely lost their power for evil. It will be noticed that the times of exposure to either air or light were less than would suffice for the drying and pulverisation of the sputum under ordinary circumstances. Specimens of the same tuberculous material gave tubercle to guinea-pigs, after it had been kept in the dark, and with very little air, for 35 days. These tests were much more severe also than would be found in the case of infection to human beings. The animals employed are the most susceptible to the disease that could be found, and they took the virus through inoculation, and not merely by breathing; the usual safeguards against infection by the latter route, therefore, were entirely absent; and human beings are usually much less vulnerable by the bacillus than either guinea-pigs or rabbits. It is evident then that the virus of tubercle is readily disinfected by natural agents, such as fresh air and light, and this conclusion is strengthened by the universal testimony to the value of free ventilation and light for the prevention of the disease. General sanitary measures, therefore, directed to these ends will certainly be of great use in any attempt to stamp out the disease. Good drainage of the soil is also very effective in the same direction. It has been amply shown that drying of the subsoil in many cases takes away half the strength of the virus. I need only cite the

---

[1] *Proceedings of the Royal Society*, vol. LVI. p. 51.

observations of Dr Bowditch and Dr Buchanan on this point—observations that have been fully corroborated by the Registrar-General for Scotland, by Mr Haviland, and by myself[1].

3. The careful inspection of cowsheds, the thorough cooking of meat, and the sterilisation of milk will easily prevent the bacillus from entering the body by the alimentary canal; and the disinfection of sputum, the prevention of the formation of tuberculous dust, and the proper control of all places of public assembly will effectually prevent its entrance by the lungs.

4. We may add that the causes of bodily predisposition to phthisis are even more easily dealt with than those that exist in the case of leprosy. It is, therefore, only necessary to press forward the general sanitary measures that are concerned with these several objects, and we may regard as no Utopian dream the forecast that after only a few more years we may see the total extinction of tubercle in our land. Few people know how far we have progressed in this direction. At the commencement of this volume (facing p. 1) I have given a Chart (which has been kindly verified by Dr Tatham) showing the phthisis rate, per 10,000 of the population, during the last 75 years. It has been now brought up to date. In the year 1838 it stood at the enormous figure of over 38, and in 1894, little more than half a century later, it was only 13·8—little more than one-third of its former prevalence. A straight line, drawn from its highest to its lowest points, shows also that its decline had been remarkably steady and generally regular[2]. If phthisis were to continue to diminish in prevalence at the same increasing rate of decline for another 30 years it would then have entirely disappeared. The first great drop in its rate took place in the decade 1840–50, about the time that serious attention began to be given to sanitary

---

[1] *The Milroy Lectures for* 1890, Smith, Elder and Co., p. 44; and *Treatment of Phthisis*, same publishers, p. 61.

[2] My friend Dr Venn points out that the fact that the line joining these two points is approximately straight, and not a hyperbola, demonstrates further that the rate of diminution in the disease is an increasing one. If the percentage of diminution had remained constant during these years the fall would have been more gradual and the extinction of the disease would have been postponed indefinitely.

reforms, and especially to land drainage. It then remained scarcely reduced for about 17 years; but from 1867 to 1894 it has been steadily on the decline. It is in this period that most of the great sanitary works have been carried out in this country. Can we doubt that it is to them that we owe so substantial a diminution of the disease? And need we despair of carrying it on to its fitting close? Let it be remembered that this improvement has taken place in spite of the increasing aggregation of the population in towns, and without any special measures of repression having been attempted. It is, indeed, only recently that tubercle has been reckoned amongst preventable diseases, and although some slight efforts at the disinfection of sputum and the cleansing of rooms occupied by phthisical patients have been made, we certainly cannot ascribe any part of the improvement that has taken place to these causes[1]. What may we not hope for when these measures come to be recognised as a part of the duty of every sanitary authority throughout the kingdom[2]? It is interesting to note that the other tuberculous diseases—such as scrofula, mesenteric disease, and tuberculous meningitis—have not diminished in like proportion.

Dr Tatham has kindly sent me the following table from his decennial supplement, not yet published, from which it will be seen how slight a change has taken place in the rates of these diseases in the last 30 years. I have marked on the Chart II (b) on the opposite page the annual rates per 1,000,000 for the last 30 years.

[1] A talented writer, Mr G. Archdall Reid, in a recent work on *The Present Evolution of Man* (Chapman and Hall, 1896, pp. 279–286), ascribes the lower rate of mortality from tuberculosis amongst the British races to an increased resistance to the microbe, a power due to "the accumulation of inborn variations"; but this explanation will surely not apply to so rapid a decline as the diminution of from 60 to 70 per cent. in the course of 60 years. It is far more likely to be due to the causes to which we have assigned it: to the sanitary measures, including improved diet, which have at once and directly diminished the infecting power of the bacillus and increased the bodily powers of resistance in the mass of the population.

[2] We may, perhaps, find an additional feature of likeness between leprosy and tubercle in the fact that they have both given way, not to intentional measures of repression, but to general reforms in sanitation, by which the whole physical welfare of the nation has been raised.

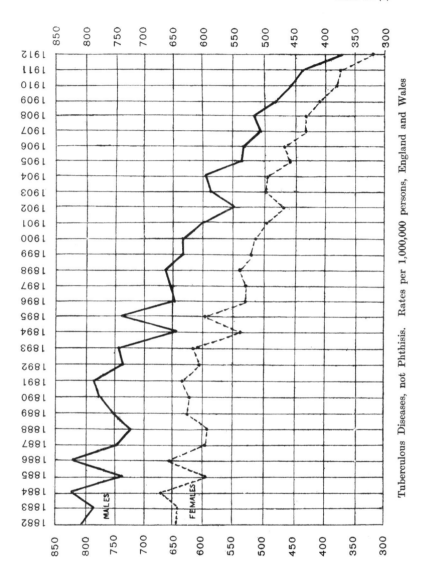

Chart *II* (b)

Tuberculous Diseases, not Phthisis. Rates per 1,000,000 persons, England and Wales

Annual Mortality per Million Living from Tuberculous
Diseases, other than Phthisis

Decennia					Rates per million
1861–70	..	..	..	..	765
1871–80	..	..	..	..	747
1881–90	..	..	..	..	696

The only possible sources of fallacy that can be discovered in these figures are (1) the uncertainty of diagnosis in the earlier periods of the registration of the causes of death, and (2) the acknowledged longer duration of phthisis in the later years. If in former days more cases of bronchitis or broncho-pneumonia were mistaken for phthisis, then these mistaken cases might have raised the apparent rates of mortality of this disease. Again, in more recent years the extension of the average duration of its progress before it ended in death would for a time postpone the appearance of these deaths in the register and would by so much lessen the phthisis rate without necessarily diminishing the real prevalence of the disease throughout the country. It is probable, however, that neither of these intrusive faults would account for the remarkably steady fall in the rate. Phthisis is a disease so easily recognised in its later stages that it has probably been reported with a fair degree of accuracy all through the period in question, and sooner or later most of the chronic cases of phthisis would have found their way into the death-roll. There is thus no important bar to our hope of a speedy extinction of phthisis if not of other tuberculous diseases, and the prophecy drawn from the analogy of leprosy is already in process of being fulfilled.

(3) THE PROSPECT OF ABOLISHING TUBERCULOSIS

TRANSACTIONS OF THE EPIDEMIOLOGICAL SOCIETY, 1899

AT the outset of the campaign about to be undertaken by the new Society for the Prevention of Tuberculosis, it is important to all who are interested in the public health that the ground to be covered should be carefully surveyed ; that we should reconnoitre the forces opposed to us ; that we should know accurately what allies, and what circumstances, are likely to help us, and discover what steps should be taken in order to secure a successful issue. When this has been done, we may perhaps be in a position to calculate the chance of abolishing this terrible disease.

In the present paper I propose to open a discussion on all the points mentioned, and I hope to elicit opinions from the members of this important Society which will greatly forward the object we all have in view, and which will materially assist the operations of the new crusade against tubercle.

A. *The Extent of the Undertaking*

The first part of the work has necessarily to do with figures, and these at present can hardly be said to lead us as far as we could wish. We know fairly well that the disease is almost ubiquitous ; that, at any rate, it exists everywhere throughout this country ; and that it is especially prevalent where large bodies of people are massed together. But we have to deal with the past as well as the present, and we have no figures of any value that take us back more than about 40 years.

The Registrar-General's tables commenced in the year 1838. It is difficult, however, to assign to any of them their right value. There must have been errors in diagnosis in the past, as there are now, and it is not certain that our forefathers made more mistakes than do the present generation of medical practitioners. There was then, as there is now, the tendency on the one hand to exaggerate the nature of the disease which has caused death, and to make it appear that death was inevitable ; and on the other hand,

there was the reluctance to place a stigma upon a family escutcheon
by writing down the name of what was considered to be an hereditary disease. Perhaps these two opposing sources of fallacy may
to some extent balance one another, and the final result may
approximate to the truth ; but in some parts of the country
there is another still more serious cause of error, namely, the
registration of uncertified deaths by relatives ; and in Wales
nearly very illness accompanied by wasting is put down by these
persons as due to consumption. Yet the figures, as they stand,
must be taken for what they are worth, for they are our only means
of appreciating the extent of the disease, both now and in the past.
Moreover, we may remember the wonderful accuracy of many of
the late Sir W. Farr's deductions from statistics which were even
more imperfect than these. Fortunately, the figures are of such
a nature as to override the possibility that our conclusions could
be materially affected by errors in one direction or another. I
have already called attention to them, in a comparison between
tuberculosis and leprosy[1]. See Chart I (facing p. 1).

From that Chart it will be seen that there has been an
almost steady decline in the former disease—tuberculosis—in this
country, since the date of the first records of the Registrar-General
in the year 1838.

In the year 1838 the phthisis-rate stood at the enormous figure of
over 3800 per million of population; but in 1896, it was only 1305 :
about one-third of its former fatality. A straight line drawn from the
highest to the lowest point shows how steady and regular has been
its decline. If phthisis were to continue to decrease at the same
increasing rate of diminution for another 30 years, it would then
have entirely disappeared. When the rate of mortality from
phthisis is broken up into groups at the different ages, a still more
striking picture of its tendency to disappear is given.

It has been possible to make this calculation since the year
1861 ; and in the last return of the Registrar-General, Dr Tatham
gives a very interesting Table (p. xxvi), which is well worth trans-
cribing.

From this Table (I) it would appear that phthisis has diminished

---

[1] *The Lancet*, July 11, 1896.

especially among women, who were at one time the most frequent victims to the disease : " the decrease among males and among females being equal to 40 and 54 per cent. respectively."

TABLE I.—*Mortality from Phthisis in Groups of Ages,* 1861–96
(*Per Million at each Age*)

	Periods	All Ages	0–	5–	10–	15–	20–	25–	35–	45–	55–	65–	75–
Males	1861–70	2467	990	431	605	2190	3883	4094	4116	3861	3297	2024	65
	1871–80	2209	783	310	481	1675	3092	3699	4120	3860	3195	1925	60
	1881–90	1847	553	253	342	1287	2333	3024	3562	3488	2916	1816	68
	1891–95	1633	467	197	260	1076	2026	2548	3268	3205	2687	1572	56
	1896	1485	392	150	203	913	1848	2285	3029	3043	2599	1329	51
Females	1861–70	2483	947	477	1045	3112	3967	4378	3900	2850	2965	1239	44
	1871–80	2028	750	375	846	2397	3140	3543	3401	2464	1777	1093	40
	1881–90	1609	518	327	699	1800	2315	2787	2730	2053	1512	974	39
	1891–95	1303	421	260	561	1428	1740	2155	2305	1742	1294	800	35
	1896	1138	349	204	454	1183	1562	1874	2090	1543	1170	676	37

When we take the middle period of life only, the diminution which has taken place in the last 35 years is still more striking. At the several ages, from 15 to 35, in the decade 1861–70, the rates for males were 2190, 3883, and 4094. In 1896 the corresponding figures were 913, 1848, and 2285 : only about one-half (49·7 per cent.) of the phthisis-rates 30 years before.

Among females, the figures in 1861–70 at the same ages, were, 3112, 3967, and 4378 ; whilst in 1896 they were respectively 1183, 1562, and 1874 : a still greater diminution of three-fifths in the 30 years (59·6 per cent.).

In Table II, Dr Tatham has also kindly calculated for me the rates per million at the age-group 15 to 35 years.

TABLE II. *Mortality from Phthisis, in England and Wales, at the Age-Group* 15–35 *Years*

	Periods	Deaths	Mean Population	Phthisis Death-Rate per Million
Males	1861–70	118,628	3,420,172	3468
	1896	8,939	5,099,363	1753
Females	1861–70	144,780	3,701,738	3911
	1896	8,745	5,494,377	1592

These figures only confirm the previous calculation.

The saving of life from this destroying agent alone, in the last 50 years, must therefore be enormous.

The conclusion to be drawn from these figures is that, within the period in question, conditions must have been introduced into the lives of the people which are hostile to the bacillus of tubercle, and which are therefore working in our favour.

It would not be difficult to single out some of the favouring circumstances which have conduced to this astonishing reduction in the rate of mortality from phthisis. I think that it will be granted at once that none of the sources of fallacy before mentioned can account for it. It is most probable that it has been due to the great changes in the conditions of life which have taken place within the present century ; and especially to the attention which, during the reign of Queen Victoria, has been paid to questions of public health.

It may be observed on consulting Chart I, facing p. 1, that the first great drop in the phthisis-rate took place in the decade 1840–50, about the time that serious attention began to be given to sanitary reforms, and especially to *land-drainage*. It then remained scarcely reduced for about 17 years ; but from 1867 to 1896 the decrease of the disease has been continuous. It is in this period that most of the great sanitary works have been carried out in this country. We can hardly doubt that it is to them that we owe so substantial a diminution of the disease. We must also give some credit to the higher standard of living among the working classes, to the better and more abundant food, the warmer or more suitable clothing, and above all to the improved dwellings, which have now been built in all our towns for the accommodation of artizans and labourers[1].

On the other hand, it certainly cannot be ascribed to any special measures of repression against the disease. It has taken place without any attempts at disinfection, or destruction, of the *materies morbi*, and in spite of the increasing aggregation of the population within the areas of our manufacturing towns.

It will be necessary presently to inquire more closely into the

---

[1] The fact that women have been the chief beneficiaries points to this last-named circumstance as the chief agent in relief, seeing that females are, for the most part, the keepers at home.

several circumstances which enhance or diminish the virulence of the bacillus of tubercle ; but it is desirable first to estimate the extent to which tuberculosis at present prevails.

In order to ascertain this, we have to return to the Registrar-General's figures. In the year 1896 he tells us that there were 40,251 deaths from phthisis, and 19,040 deaths from other tubercular diseases—in all nearly 60,000 deaths from this disorder.

If we accept the estimate of the average duration of phthisis, which has been made by such competent observers as Drs C. T. Williams, James Pollock, and others, at something over four years, we shall have to conclude that over 160,000 consumptives, and perhaps 30,000 or 40,000 persons affected by other tubercular disorders, are now existing in England and Wales ; in all about 200,000 persons who are capable of producing the material of the disease ; and, if we include Scotland and Ireland, probably not fewer than 300,000 persons are thus affected within the British Isles at the present time. But even this vast army of sufferers hardly represents the whole force which we have to control, and to prevent from spreading the disease, for there are certainly many thousands of others who are as yet unconscious of its presence, but who are nevertheless capable of doing mischief.

We are told by many eminent pathologists that from 20 to 30 per cent. of all persons dying in hospitals between the ages of 25 and 75 show signs of healed tubercular lesions. Many of these patients had never been made aware of their condition ; and there must be a multitude of others in whom the disease has not yet been detected, who are only waiting to join the ranks of those who are already enrolled, and who are even now as dangerous as our more open enemies.

Last, and probably not least, if we are to take account of all possible sources of tuberculous virus, we must not forget the hundreds of thousands of cattle, and other animals, which are affected with tubercular disease, which are daily spreading it about broadcast, and which are even less under control in this respect than human beings. It has been pointed out also that most of the animals in our zoological gardens are tuberculous ; and, although avian tubercle is supposed to be incapable of infecting the higher orders of animals, Prof. Nocard, of Alfort, has recently shown that, under certain conditions, the virus is capable of modification, so as to become a source of danger.

B. *The Sources of the Strength and Weakness of the Bacillus*

In these days of bacteriological research there is nothing wonderful in the fact that so small a cause as a tiny vegetable mould can produce such a vast amount of evil. It is one of the " weak things of the world " which the Almighty has chosen " to confound the things which are mighty " ; and we may perhaps be allowed to surmise that its action is permitted in order to bring men to a knowledge of His beneficent " Laws of Health." At all events, its activity has had this result ; and in any case we are bound to search for the sources of its great power for evil. These are:

1. *The immense number of the enemy.* Tuberculous patients are to be found in all communities of men, and the amount of virulent material which is dispersed by them is probably enormous. It has been calculated that about two millions of bacilli are often contained in a single portion of sputum, expelled from the lungs of a tuberculous person.

2. *The tenacity of life of the bacillus under certain favourable conditions.* I have myself found that it retains its virulence for three months, when kept in a small insanitary cottage in Ancoats ; and other observers have recorded much longer periods of infectiveness. Under these unhealthy conditions, tuberculous sputum has been found to resist all the changes of the seasons : wetness, dryness, freezing, considerable heat, snow, rain and hail.

I have also found that the bacillus will grow upon pure filter-paper, if kept saturated with organically-charged fluids, condensed from the vapour of ground air, from healthy and diseased breath, from humidified weaving sheds, and from cellars.

3. *The contamination of milk by tuberculous material.* This is another important source of infection, and meat and other kinds of food are probably sometimes media for conveying the disease.

4. *The chronic character of the complaint.* This is itself a powerful influence in its favour. It prevents the early recognition of the disease ; it permits a dangerous kind of intercourse with other individuals : especially when the affected person indulges in the filthy habit of expectorating in an unhealthy dwelling, or

in an ill-ventilated workshop, thus facilitating the constant and long-continued manufacture of tuberculous dust, and so endangering the lives of his companions and fellow-workpeople.

5. *The long incubation period of the disease.* This often prevents the source of infection from being recognised, and, its origin being thus concealed, measures for preventing its spread to others cannot be undertaken until it is too late.

6. *The habit of the specific microbe of contracting alliances* with other organisms, such as the tetragonus, streptococci and staphylococci. This habit enhances its power for evil, both by increasing the fatality of the disease, and by preparing the way for its entrance into the human body.

7. *The power possessed by the bacillus of producing " toxines."* This probably helps somewhat in the same direction as the habit just mentioned.

8. *The readiness with which the complaint can be transferred to cattle,* and to other domesticated animals. This increases the scope of its action.

9. *Lastly, the failure of ordinary disinfectants to kill the microbe.* This increases the difficulty of dealing with it.

It will be seen, therefore, that small though it be, we have no insignificant foe to meet ; yet, on the other hand, there is no need to despair of successfully coping with it.

In the great discussion on tuberculosis, in the year 1885, Dr Moxon[1] made the striking remark that " The life of the bacillar parasite is difficult, easily discouraged by unfavourable circumstances, like an aphis by an easterly wind " ; and I think we shall find that his statement is strictly in accordance with the facts.

There are many conditions adverse to the bacillus of tubercle ; otherwise we may be sure that, without special measures of repression, it would hardly have given ground, as we have seen that it has done. Some of them may be briefly considered :

1. *The bacillus has a constant tendency to lose virulence,* and even to decline in the vigour of its growth. Under circumstances most favourable to its longevity, it usually diminishes in power ; and, unless it is passed through the bodies of animals, it cannot be made to retain its virulence. I am informed that most of the

---

[1] *British Medical Journal,* 1885, vol. i. p. 130.

specimens which are to be found in our bacteriological laboratories are non-virulent. The successive cultures gradually lose their strength ; and even simple keeping, under favourable circumstances, will not preserve their properties.

2. *It is extremely susceptible to the action of sunlight and air,* in spite of its resistance to certain of the meteorological influences which have been already mentioned.

In a research devoted to this subject by Prof. Delépine and myself, in one series of trials, all the experiments[1] showed that very short exposures to sunlight and air sufficed to deprive the organism, even in sputum, of all virulence. In one case[2], a specimen exposed to light and air for two days only, with but little radiant sunshine, was found to have entirely lost its power for evil. Another specimen, exposed for three days, with only one hour of sunshine, gave a similar result[3].

Ventilation alone, in the dark, also diminishes, though it does not necessarily destroy, virulence[4].

It is important to notice that, in all the experiments on light and air, the times of exposure ascertained to be sufficient to disinfect the temporary habitat of the bacillus were less than would suffice for the pulverisation of the sputum, under ordinary circumstances ; yet specimens of the same sputum gave tubercle to guinea-pigs after it had been kept in the dark, with little air, for 30 days. *In other words, virulent tuberculous dust cannot be formed in well-lighted, well-ventilated places.*

Sunlight and air are probably the most powerful disinfectants known of the material of tuberculosis.

3. *Fortunately, man is one of the animals refractory to the action of the bacillus.* In man, when infection takes place through the skin, the poison is usually arrested at the first lymphatic gland, and is then often discharged from the body by suppuration. When the virus makes its entrance by the respiratory tract, it is highly probable that it cannot take root, unless some previous injury has afforded it a resting-place, or some abrasion has given it an entrance into the system.

---

[1] *Researches on Tuberculosis*, the Weber-Parkes Prize Essay for 1897, Smith, Elder and Co., pp. 21–22.   [2] *Loc. cit.* Table XIII, No. 190.
[3] *Loc. cit.* Table XIII, No. 156.   [4] *Loc cit.* pp. 18–19.

4. *The long period of incubation,* though it disguises the source of infection, is yet an important safeguard to the individual. No infection from tuberculosis can take place unless the bodily tissues are in such a condition as to receive, and to nourish into colonies, the bacilli which have found an entrance. This condition is usually the result of some state of the bodily constitution, due to some predisposing injury, or some weakness, hereditary or acquired.

In a perfectly healthy human body, there are a multitude of barriers against the establishment of colonies of the bacillus, barriers which are hardly ever entirely overcome. Amongst the more important of these defences may be mentioned : (1) the aqueous vapour of the breath, which entangles all solid particles in its meshes and deposits them in the glairy mucus lining of the air-passages ; (2) the continual working of this mucus, by the currents of air, and by the action of the " cilia " lining the air-channels, towards the mouth ; (3) the presence of protecting glands extending from the throat to distant ramifications of the bronchial tubes ; (4) the action of aggressive warrior elements, the " phagocyte " cells.

The so-called " giant cells " have apparently this function ; and it is tolerably certain that there are other cells in the lymphatic glands, and in other parts, whose office it is to seek for and to devour intruding bacilli and other organisms.

5. *Koch's discovery of " tuberculin."* As a test for the presence of tubercle, this will certainly in the future be of enormous service in assisting us to stamp out this disease in cattle.

6. *The drying of the subsoil.* The influence of this upon the prevalence of phthisis is as yet imperfectly understood ; but no doubt can now be entertained that thorough drainage and drying of the soil are important agents in preventing the disease.

There are many other influences—some hostile, others predisposing, to tuberculosis. Among the latter we may place hereditary weaknesses of certain organs of the body, especially of the lungs, which produce susceptibility to contract the disease, and increase the tendency to a rapid and fatal issue. It is well known also that there are certain disorders which leave behind them similar proclivities ; such complaints, for instance, as enteric fever, measles, and others, which are likely to end in permanent disablement of portions of lung tissue. Other affections, tending to general debility, are likewise favourable to tuberculosis, such as diabetes, syphilis, alcoholism, cancer ; and pregnancy seems in some persons to have the same effect. Susceptibility to tubercle is often acquired by persons who have suffered from other diseases of the lungs and pleura ; or from external injuries affecting the joints, the skin, or other parts of the body.

Broncho-pneumonia and cirrhosis of the lungs, arising from inhaling irritating dusts, are peculiarly likely to lead to the further deposit of tubercular material, as the bacilli often inspired along with the dust find suitable resting-places within the damaged tissues.

When we add to these conditions, so favourable to the enemy, the existence of overcrowded, unwholesome dwellings, of work-shops insufficiently supplied with air and light, of theatres and other places of public assembly badly ventilated, and seldom visited by rays of sunlight, we shall not have much difficulty in accounting for the differences in rates of mortality from consumption and other forms of tubercular disease.

There are whole areas of insanitary houses, in most of our large towns, where the disease prevails three or four times as much as in the more healthy districts; and it is sadly interesting to compare the incidence of phthisis upon the classes of workpeople employed in trades where the ventilation of workshops is not compulsory, with the relative immunity of those to whom plenty of air is supplied.

C. *The Prospect of Victory*

This brief review of the opposing forces may perhaps enable us to form some idea of the way in which the campaign now opening will end. In the first place, it is of happy augury for the result of the contest that our enemy is at present in full retreat. It is well known that a campaign which begins with victory is often carried out by the victor with great advantage. The common phrase that " nothing succeeds like success " tritely expresses this fact. But, in the present case, the dispersal of a large contingent of the army of tubercular disease should do something more than

animate us for the final contest.   It points the way to further
victory.

We have already seen that the great and steady decline in
the phthisis-rate coincides in point of time with the introduction
of measures of sanitary reform, and with the improvement in the
general conditions of life which have taken place during the reign
of Queen Victoria : it cannot be traced to any special measures
of repression, such as isolation of phthisical persons, or disinfection
of sputum, or of houses.   Surely it should encourage us to put in
the forefront of the coming battle all the means which have already
proved so successful.

(a) It is imperative, therefore, that all sanitary authorities
should put in force the manifold powers which they now possess
for improving the public health ; not only that they should attend
to the sewerage, and house and subsoil drainage, but that they
should turn their attention to the still more important question of
removing from their streets and dwellings and places of social
assembly, the more subtle and even more dangerous " air-sewage."
Owing to the prevalence of the disease among cattle also, similar
measures will have to be taken with regard to cow-sheds, etc.

Viewed in relation to our present subject, the prevention of
phthisis, the problem of removing organic impurities from the air
we breathe is a very wide and difficult one.   It involves not only
the admission, without draught, of a certain number of cubic feet
of air to living rooms or to places where human beings congregate,
but that the air so admitted should be itself fairly pure.

It is important, doubtless, that all insanitary property should
either be destroyed or made fit for healthy habitation ; and that
back-to-back houses, undrained and unaerated basement dwellings,
should be done away with ; that workshops and factories should be
efficiently ventilated ; that schools and places of public assembly
should be more fully supplied with a flow of air adequate to the
needs of their temporary inmates.   But all this will be of comparatively little use if the outer air be in such a condition as to induce
all cleanly people to close their windows against it.

The outer air must therefore be kept as pure as possible ; in
the streets, free course must be given to the wind ; there must be
no blind alleys or streets closed at one end ; and, wherever

possible, the width of streets must be proportional to the height of buildings, and an adequate space must be left around each building. By this means both sufficient air and sufficient light may have access to the dwellings, and the air will be freed from much of its impurity.

Local authorities, therefore, will have to put in force their strongest powers for the prevention of pollution of the air, by smoke and noxious vapours ; they must provide ample lung-space in the shape of public parks and open playgrounds ; and they will have to carry out extensive works of reconstruction of insanitary areas.

Building byelaws must be carefully scrutinised, and if necessary amended, and the various " Rookeries " Acts must be ruthlessly put in force. When all this is done, we cannot doubt that the great shrinkage in the mass of tubercular disease will continue to go on. I am the more anxious to emphasise this point, because it seems to me that most of the anti-tubercle societies are inclined to neglect this vital subject, for disinfection and other matters of somewhat less importance.

(*b*) In the next place, if, by means of disinfection of sputum and destruction of tuberculous dust in dwellings, and places of public assembly, we cut off the supplies of infectious material, the assault of the enemy must fail for want of ammunition. Let it be clearly understood, however, what is involved in this method of carrying on the war. It will be necessary to bring into action all the time-honoured machinery of notification, disinfection, isolation (in certain cases), and hospital accommodation.

(*c*) *Notification.* It is important that the full extent of the attacking force should be known. There is an "intelligence department" in every army.

It is essential, therefore, that every case of tuberculosis, as soon as its nature and locality are known, should be notified to the Medical Officer of Health in every district. It does not follow that any immediate action should be taken by him. We are told by Dr Hermann Biggs that, in New York, cases in private houses, and under the care of private physicians, are not in any way interfered with. " The data regarding such cases are recorded, but they are not visited by the inspectors of the Department ; no circulars of information are sent to them, nor are they interfered with in any way, except by special request of the attending physician. The Department has always fully recognised the importance of non-intervention between the physician and his patient in tuberculosis, in cases in which the intelligent practitioner may be trusted to give the simple instructions necessary to prevent the transmission of the disease to others."

In that city, however, " cases of tuberculosis, reported to the Department by the public institutions of the city, are visited at their houses by medical inspectors, specially detailed for the purpose, who give verbal directions respecting the proper care of the sputum, and leave circulars of direction. Cases requiring hospital treatment are visited by a special inspector, who examines the patient, and collects some of his sputum, which is afterwards examined in the laboratories of the Department."

If tubercle bacilli are found, and the patient is undoubtedly tuberculous, and is not in circumstances to receive proper care and medical attendance, or is a source of danger to others, and desires hospital treatment, he or she is removed, by order of the Department, to one of two specially designated hospitals.

I have described the New York method of notification and its sequences thus at length, because it seems to be worthy of careful consideration. It affords intelligence of all overt cases of the disease, and yet is followed by action only in those cases where such action seems needful for the protection of the rest of the community.

(*d*) *Disinfection*, either under the guidance of the regular medical attendant, or of the Medical Officer of Health, is the natural sequence of notification. There are published many admirable leaflets of directions how to deal with tuberculous material : these will have to be distributed to every house inhabited by a consumptive or tuberculous patient. The dwellings of such persons will have to be thoroughly disinfected by Professor Delépine's methods, sometimes during the life of the patient, always after the removal to other quarters, and after death.

(*e*) *Isolation* may be necessary in the case of unteachable persons, or where there is such destitution that the proper precautions cannot be carried out. For this purpose—

(*f*) *Hospital accommodation* will be required. At the present time, in most parts of England, such accommodation is only afforded by the workhouse authorities ; but I would submit that it would be a legitimate expenditure on the part of local boards of health if they were to provide male and female wards for the reception of such cases, in connection with their hospitals for infectious diseases.

(*g*) There is yet another very important weapon in our armoury for the abatement of tubercular disease, and that is the *abolition of the complaint* in our herds of cattle. It is doubtless true that if all milk were boiled and all meat thoroughly well cooked, there would be little danger of contracting disease by the medium of the articles of food ; but this precaution would not obviate the risk of infection from the tuberculous material scattered about the byres by the cattle themselves. Moreover, who is to make sure that the precaution is always carried out ? There will always be careless people who will not take the necessary trouble, and there are many children who will not take boiled milk.

The only way of avoiding all these dangers is to form herds of tubercle-free cows. As Bang, in Denmark, has shown, it is quite possible, without much expense, to extinguish the disease within the generation of cattle which it affects : " provided sufficient means are taken to protect the succeeding generation from becoming affected."

The same object has been attained more rapidly in England, notably by Lord Vernon, of Sudbury. It needs, therefore, only a strong effort so to influence public opinion that the use of tuberculin, as a test, should become general throughout the country, and that all herds of cattle should be rendered innocuous to the public health.

It is evident from the foregoing facts, in the first place, that the forces opposed to us are steadily on the decline ; and that this diminution in the disease must be attributed to the inherent weakness of the microbe, as compared with the powerful influence of ordinary sanitary reforms, without special measures of repression ; and, in the second place, that we possess in disinfection, in the tuberculin test, etc., potent weapons of precision, with which,

when fully put into action, we may fairly hope to accomplish the
final conquest of the foe.

The question naturally arises, When may we expect complete
success ?   When will tuberculosis cease out of the land ?

Judging from the past, I think that we may look for this
consummation before very long, and without waiting for a Utopian
state of things.   Already the rate of diminution in the prevalence
of phthisis is greater than that of leprosy, when that disease began
to decline.   It took at least 200 years for leprosy to diminish to any appreciable extent ; but 60 years has marked a decline
in phthisis of at least two-thirds.   When all our forces are brought
fully into action, we may surely expect that at least as great a
rate of decline will be continued ; and, in this case, another 30
years should see its vanishing point.

We can hardly doubt that the retreat will go on at an increasing
speed.   When all health authorities perform efficiently the several
tasks which have now been set before them ; when, by the means
which have been mentioned, tuberculous cattle have been abolished from our herds ; when the general public have been fully
instructed how to deal with tuberculous material ; and when,
by means of " open-air sanatoria " in connection with all our great
towns, the existing consumptives, and other tuberculous patients,
are provided with the requisite essentials for their cure, then may
we hope for complete success.

Let us take, then, for our motto, " Victoria, et per Victoriam,
Vita."

(4) THE PUBLIC-HOUSE AS A SOURCE OF PHTHISIS

MEDICAL CHRONICLE, *May*, 1904

THE influence of intemperance as a source of moral and social evil has long been a subject attracting the attention of philanthropists. Its effect in raising the " death-toll " of the United Kingdom has also been estimated by several statisticians. In a paper read before the Church of England Temperance Society (Hope Hall, Liverpool, January 25, 1878) " On the Relations between Intemperance and the Rate of Mortality," I have myself made what I considered to be a moderate estimate of the mortality due to intemperance at between 40,000 and 50,000 a year.

Attempts have moreover been made to ascertain its specific influence upon several diseases, including phthisis, but I am not aware that any definite statement was made as to the influence of the public-house upon this malady until Dr Niven approached the subject in a paper on " The Relation of Phthisis to Factory and Workshop Conditions," read at a meeting of the British Medical Association, in Manchester, in August, 1902. This paper seems to be so important that I venture now to give a brief résumé of it and to call special attention to its conclusions.

It is true that the public-house, as an infecting agent, had been grouped with other places of public resort by various writers, but, in this paper, Dr Niven brought a special indictment against the public-house as a source of phthisis, supporting his accusation not only by statistics but by observations conducted by his excellent staff of Corporation officers.

The comparative phthisis-rates of males and females, given by the Registrar-General in " Lowe's Tables," had indeed already pointed to some influence, other than merely the conditions of work, as factors in this mortality. Thus, as shown in my Milroy Lectures of 1890, the high phthisis-rates of males in such country places as Bury St Edmunds, Cambridge, Brighton and Salisbury, and the low phthisis-rates of women could hardly be accounted for by the occupation of males and females in these places.

Again, in the adjoining Chart II (*c*), which I have drawn from the interesting tables given by Dr Tatham in the last report of the Registrar-General, it will be seen that, in the last 20 years, though the phthisis-rate has gone down for both males and females, the male-rate is still the higher, and has been much the slower in its descent. Seeing that the other conditions of life must have exerted similar influences on both sexes, it seems probable that frequency of resort to the public-house, on the part of the males, may have had something to do with the abiding differences in the rates of the two sexes.

I have appended to this Chart another (Chart II *b*) drawn from the same sources, giving the mortality variations, during the same period, of other tuberculous diseases, not phthisis. From this it will be seen that, while this mortality slightly diminishes in both sexes, the male death-rate descends even more rapidly than the female ; showing that the improvement in the home conditions of life had had at least as great an influence upon males as upon females, in preserving them from these diseases, and that thus we must look for some condition outside the home that was favourable to the spread of phthisis among males. That this outside influence had something to do with a difference in the drinking habits of the two sexes is probable, and a consideration of the state of most public-houses adds to this probability.

The public-house, viewed from a sanitary point of view, is certainly an object of suspicion as an infective centre. It not only shares the likelihood of tuberculous contamination with other places of public assembly, but has special dangers of its own. Its bars and taprooms are usually dark, dirty and ill-ventilated. They are often overcrowded, especially in the evening, by crowds of workmen and loungers, many of them consumptives. These people spit freely both into the spittoons, containing sawdust or sand, and on to the floor. The floors are for the most part covered with dry sand or sawdust, and are only swept occasionally, perhaps once or twice a week. The sputum from their occupants, much of it charged with virulent tubercular material, is mixed with the sand or sawdust ; it is dried up and ground into fine powder under the heels of the drinkers. When it is swept up, some of it flies into the air, and floats there on delicate wings of mucus or

Chart II (c)

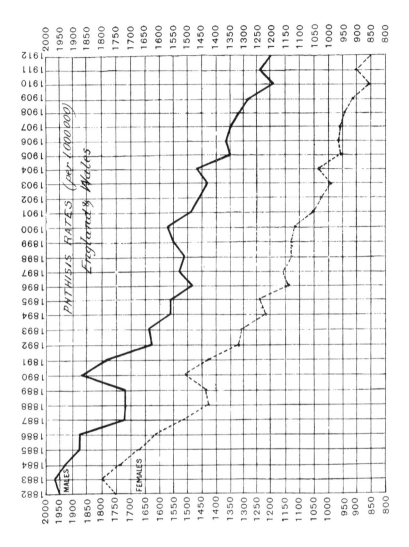

PHTHISIS RATES (per 1,000,000)
England & Wales

Chart II (b)

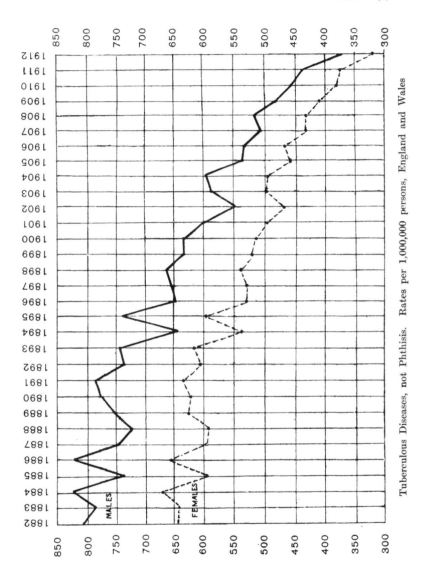

Tuberculous Diseases, not Phthisis.   Rates per 1,000,000 persons, England and Wales

epithelial scales. It is thus capable of being conveyed into the lungs of susceptible persons, and of transmitting the disease. Add to all this risk the probability that spray from the coughing of some consumptive may also pass into the air breathed by others, and we cannot be surprised that tuberculous infection arises from this source. I have ascertained that, at any rate in a large proportion of public-houses, the unwholesome conditions above described are present and that the account of the modes of cleansing these places is not overstated.

In order to determine the part played by the public-house in causing the excessive mortality from phthisis among males, Dr Niven enters upon an intricate inquiry, the details of which are given in the paper above mentioned. He shows first that there is no special proclivity to the disease in males. Thus : (*a*) in 19 out of 44 counties, the female phthisis-rate exceeds the male, *i.e.* in most of the agricultural and coal-mining districts ; (*b*) the rate, at the earlier " age-periods," shows no undue incidence upon the male sex, but rather the contrary. It is only at the later ages, between 35 and 45, that males begin to die of phthisis at a greater rate than females.

Dr Niven then proceeds to inquire what possible influences could be found bearing exclusively or especially upon men ? To answer this question he goes deeply into a most complex investigation. First, by means of the " Occupation Tables," given in Part ii of the Supplement to the 55th Annual Report of the Registrar-General, he obtains the comparative mortality figures for phthisis, at ages from 25 to 26, and he is thus able to pick out the trades suffering most severely from the disease, and the numbers employed in each kind of work. Excluding the uncertain group of unoccupied males, in which the mortality from phthisis is enormous, he forms three other groups each having an excessive mortality from the disease.

Group I comprises general labourers in the industrial districts, hawkers, dock and wharf labourers, messengers and porters, innkeepers and publicans and their servants. These number about 278,333·3.

Group II includes printers, tailors, shoemakers, workers in metal other than iron, cabinet-makers, wood-turners, wool, silk, etc., dyers, drapers and Manchester warehousemen, watch, clock, etc., makers. These number 402,666·6.

Group III contains workers with smaller, though still excessive, phthisis mortalities, formidable from their numbers, such as commercial clerks, coach and cab service, merchant seamen, engine, machine, etc., makers and fitters, nail, anchor and chain makers, bricklayers, masons and builders, plumbers, painters and glaziers. Number, 1,208,333·3.

Altogether nearly two million workers are included in these three groups.

Dr Niven then classifies the several factors predisposing to phthisis, such as overcrowding, dusts, insufficient nourishment, alcoholism, etc., under three heads : (1) social conditions ; (2) alcohol ; and (3) occupation. The question to be determined was the relative share, in the production of phthisis among workpeople, taken by each of these several factors. The problem was by no means easy of solution, seeing that all three groups of influences were at work at the same time. Nevertheless it had to be faced.

1. Under the head of *Social Conditions* are included such matters as poverty, unhealthy dwellings, overcrowding, bad ventilation, bad drainage, common lodging-houses and so forth. All of these undoubtedly " exercise a powerful influence on the production of phthisis," but, on the whole, it will be found that " they are inadequate, by themselves, to produce the differences between the male and female phthisis-rates, rather their tendency would be to raise the female death-rate over that of the males." The influence of the public-house and other kindred places, where the men congregate and drink, would, however, help largely to turn the scale.

2. *Alcoholism.* In order to test the influence of drink upon the production of phthisis, Dr Niven now calls attention to another table, drawn from the same source as the first, which shows the comparative mortality among the several groups of workers, from diseases presumably of alcoholic origin, such as " alcoholism, liver disease, suicide, bronchitis, pneumonia, and nervous diseases." Although there may be some doubt as to whether all of these deaths are really due to alcohol, on the whole we may generally

arrive at a conclusion as to whether alcoholism is exceptionally present in any particular occupation, by referring to the total deaths from the above-mentioned causes. From this table we see at once that all the occupations included in Group I, and also some of those in Group II, are greatly affected by alcoholic diseases. They are also, as we have seen, exceptionally affected by phthisis. Dr Niven concludes, therefore, that, to account for the prevalence of phthisis in these workpeople, " there are required two factors— intemperance and infection in inns and public-houses—infection which depends on the general habit of spitting on the floor, and which assails the persons attending upon the customers as well as the customers themselves."

3. *Occupation*. In order to estimate the degree to which the conditions of work weighed upon both males and females, and increased the tendency to phthisis, apart from the two other groups of factors, Dr Niven now entered upon a further inquiry. By means of the admirable organisation at his command in Manchester, he instituted an investigation as to the conditions of work of each class of workpeople there. He first had the phthisis death-rates for the City of Manchester calculated at six groups of ages for males and females separately for a variety of occupations, the deaths being for the three years 1899 to 1901, and the populations at groups of ages are the Census figures for 1901. This table not only gave him the opportunity of comparing the phthisis-rates of both males and females in certain groups of occupations, but by noting the ages at which the deaths occurred, it was possible to guess at the trades in which the disease was favoured by the kind of work itself, and those in which some other outside influence, like that of the public-house, was at work.

If the deaths of males and females were fairly evenly spread over the various ages, and were somewhat similar in men and women, it was reasonable to conclude that they were mainly due to the employment. or rather to the conditions under which it was carried on—to such conditions, for instance, as the want of ventilation, dusts, amount of spitting about on the floors of the workshops, etc. On the other hand, if the phthisis mortality was only excessive among males at the later ages, the source must be sought for outside the work-place. Thus, in the case of the cotton operatives, the female phthisis-rate is the greater at the ages of 15 to 25, but at every higher age-group the male rate is much in excess. In the case of tailors, in which the females enjoy no advantage in respect of ventilation or cleanliness, apart from personal habits, the female death-rate is higher at ages 15 to 25, but beyond this age-period, the male death-rate is much the higher of the two. There are, in fact, no fewer than 18 deaths from phthisis in the three years at ages 45 to 65 among 742 male tailors, and no deaths at all among 512 female tailors. The same difference is apparent among boot-makers, costermongers, hawkers, and street sellers. Dr Niven remarks " it is natural to expect that, where intemperance prevails, the females should suffer heavily from phthisis at the earlier ages, from the effects of malnutrition, and it seems difficult to avoid the conclusion that the excess of the male rates at the higher ages is largely due to intemperance.

These conclusions, from the compared male and female rates, are confirmed by noticing that the number of deaths among persons known to be given to intemperance take place mostly at the later ages. Thus law clerks have a very high phthisis-rate at ages between 25 and 45. Coachmen, cabmen, grooms, etc., messengers, porters, and watchmen also suggest a phthisis mortality due to resort to public-houses. In the case of carpenters and joiners, the suggestion is rather occupational, but in the case of bricklayers and their labourers, masons and their assistants, intemperance is strongly suggested. In inn and hotel keepers and publicans the phthisis-rates are very evenly distributed, as we should expect from their occupation. The figures for general labourers also point to some progressive influence, but, as large numbers of these live in common lodging-houses, there is no doubt direct infection is at work, and, in addition, intemperance and the public-house also play a large part in causing the excessive rates observed.

Dr Niven then gives the results of direct observation of the several conditions of life in persons notified to him as having died of phthisis. In 466 of these cases, it was possible to make some guess at the sources of infection, and in many of them this was found in the home, or in the presence of infectious dust in the places of work ; but there were also " a number of instances in which the infection appears to have been contracted in the public-house." From the cases voluntarily notified to him, Dr Niven was able to select certain occupations in which a considerable number of cases had been notified from particular factories and workshops. He and his assistant medical officers and sanitary inspectors then proceeded to visit the various works thus placed under suspicion. The homes of the individual cases concerned were visited and their histories, as regarded exposure to infection otherwise than through the workshop, were taken down; in fact, every circumstance which could be thought of as affecting the incidence of phthisis on these operatives was recorded. In many of the works, the chief factors making for phthisis observed were the great amount of dust, and the general habit of spitting amongst the male workers ; this did not happen amongst the female operatives. More dangerous even than spitting in the workshop was the expectoration which was frequently observed to have occurred in the " closets." This was again confined to the males.

We have here, therefore, in a certain number of places, a probable source of the excessive phthisis-rates among males ; but it is limited in its operation, and Dr Niven was again obliged to come to the conclusion that in some of the works, the excessive incidence of phthisis amongst the male workers was largely " due to these men frequenting public-houses, where the inhabitants of common lodging-houses and other consumptives also assembled." In fact, " at one of the works concerned, the effects of the industry could be set aside, as well as the possibility of direct infection, except perhaps in the closets." In another, there was no industrial dust, though spitting was excessive. In both, the influences of the public-house and of the dwelling could apparently be regarded as operating to a specially mischievous extent.

After enumerating a number of measures, which he regards as essential to the suppression of the disease, Dr Niven finally concludes his admirable paper by saying : " It is essential, I think, that public-houses should be placed under strict legislation in respect of cleanliness, and that spitting in public-houses should be prohibited. It is partly in the workshops, but to a much larger extent in public-houses, that the inhabitants of common lodging-houses propagate, amongst the industrial classes, the tuberculous phthisis which makes such ravages amongst them."

In a private letter which I have received from Dr Niven he thus sums up the whole question : " Alcoholism alone will not account for the male excess in phthisis. Privation will not. The excess (among males) takes place when men and women are working in adjoining rooms ; in the same building ; at the same occupations. There are two cardinal differences between men and women which we know to have a bearing upon phthisis—spitting and frequenting places where people spit (chiefly the public-house). The workshop and public-house both play their part, but especially the latter."

I have suggested to Dr Niven that it would be desirable to procure direct evidence of the infective character of the dust in public-houses, but, short of this, I think that Dr Niven's indictment against these places is fairly well proved by the circumstantial evidence which he adduces. It is on this account that I have ventured to attempt this brief summary of his important paper, and also in the hope that it will call more attention to the paper itself, with its multitude of facts and figures, than seems hitherto to have been given to it.

(5) PHTHISIS-RATES : THEIR SIGNIFICANCE AND THEIR TEACHING

TRANSACTIONS OF THE EPIDEMIOLOGICAL SOCIETY, 1904–5

STATISTICS of mortality from pulmonary tuberculosis through-out long series of years are of great importance from both their etiological and their economic bearing. Their variations in successive years throw light upon possible causes of aggravation or decline, and point the way towards the measures that should be taken for the abolition of the disease.

In the present Paper the following sources of information have been used :

Through the courtesy of Dr Tatham, of Somerset House, I have been furnished with many statistics, derived from the Returns of the Registrar-General for England and Wales, since the year 1838 ; the four years, 1843 to 1846 inclusive, being omitted, as the causes of deaths were not given during those years.

Sir Stair Agnew, the Registrar-General for Scotland, has, through Mr Hamilton, kindly provided me with the male and female phthisis-rates since the year 1871 ; and Dr Matheson, Registrar-General for Ireland, has afforded me the opportunity of obtaining similar statistics for Ireland since the year 1861.

Dr Hope, of Liverpool, Sir Shirley F. Murphy, of London, and Dr Niven, of Manchester, have given me the figures relating to these cities.

I desire to express my cordial thanks to these gentlemen for the valuable assistance which they have given to me[1].

I have projected the several sets of figures thus obtained upon the accompanying Charts, so as to show graphically their variations. The method allows us to note their rise and fall in different years, to compare the shape of their curves, their differences and their coincidences, which are thus displayed much more readily than is possible with mere lists of figures.

[1] The Editor of the *Transactions* is also indebted to Dr Hope for much assistance in securing the reproduction of all these Charts.

Chart I (facing p. 1) represents the phthisis death-rates of persons, per 10,000 of population, in England and Wales, for each year since 1838, with the exceptions already noted, from 1843 to 1846 inclusive.

Charts II (*a*), III, and IV give the male and female rates (per 1,000,000) separately: Chart II (*a*) for England and Wales, Chart III for Scotland, and Chart IV for Ireland.

Charts V and VI supply similar rates for Liverpool and Manchester.

It must, at the outset, be pointed out that purists in the matter of statistics do not regard the figures given in the earlier years of the period thus covered as trustworthy. They prefer to limit their comparisons of the death-rates from divers diseases to the years subsequent to 1867. There were undoubtedly many imperfections in the diagnosis and in the collection of these several data in the earlier years of the Registrar-General's Returns. Thus, in his Twenty-seventh Annual Report, Dr Farr mentions serious cases of fraud on the part of Registrars : " In the course of 29 years, out of a body of 2200 officers, four—for the sake of a shilling an entry—inserted long series of fictitious entries of deaths which never occurred. They invented the particulars of hundreds of deaths."

Until the year 1874, the certificate of the cause of death was not compulsory. A proportion of the deaths were not certified by legally qualified medical practitioners. Dr Farr calculated that, at one time, "in 17 per cent. of the total number of deaths, registered in England and Wales, no clue is given as to the cause of death. At one time, in South Wales, the registration books were in a state of hopeless confusion. At Llanbedr, out of 500 notices of death, 101 were certified, 399 were not ; and, at St Davids, out of the same number, only 15 were certified."

At the present time, thanks to the efforts of Dr Farr and his successors, great improvements have taken place ; but, unfortunately, even now it cannot be said that these statistics are by any means perfect ; and, in the case of many diseases, they do not permit of any sound conclusion being founded upon them as to the true causes of death.

Some use may, however, be made of very imperfect statistical

Chart II (a)

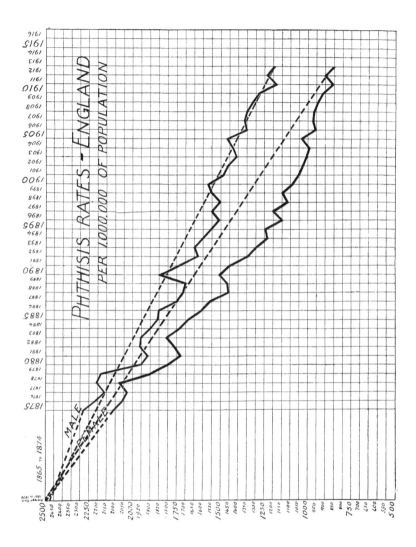

Chart III

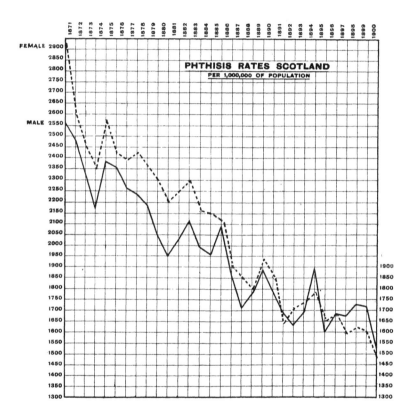

PHTHISIS RATES SCOTLAND

PER 1,000,000 OF POPULATION

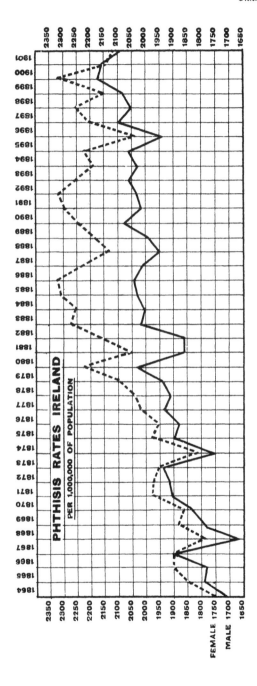

Chart IV

Chart V   *Chart VI*

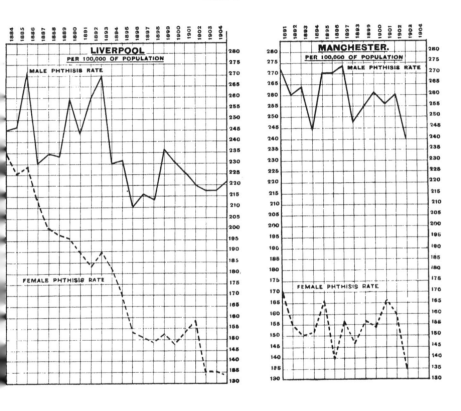

material : witness the remarkable researches of Dr William Farr himself, and of Sir John Simon.

In the case of phthisis, I am inclined to think, for the following reasons, that it is not necessary entirely to reject the mortality figures during the 30 years preceding 1868.

1. Although the early diagnosis of the disease is often difficult, it must be admitted that death from pulmonary phthisis is usually quite easy to diagnose. It will, for the most part, be correctly recorded even by unskilled persons. Most old women, in fact, could diagnose the disease in its later stages quite as well as the skilled physician.

At the outset, therefore, there is a strong probability that the registration of a death from " consumption " was genuine, even if it were only reported by relations, and not by a medical man.

2. That the earlier Returns of phthisis in the Registrar-General's Reports are probably fairly correct, is shown by their accordance with what we know of this mortality from the London Bills of Mortality. In the years 1743-53, when, as Dr Ogle says, " they were fairly accurate transcripts from the parish registers, the proportion of deaths from consumption in the Metropolis to the total deaths was rather more than one-fifth ; and, in the first Return of the Registrar-General, in 1838, in London, it was 1 to 6·8."

In other words, the rate per 1000 deaths in the former period was about 200, and in the latter about 148. Hence, in the middle of the eighteenth century, phthisis must have been still more common than in 1838 ; and thus the diminution in the mortality from the disease must have been proceeding steadily, at about the same rate as that observed in the earlier years recorded in Chart I.

3. A further proof of the sufficiently accurate character of the early returns of phthisis is to be found in the fact that, if a straight line is drawn from the lower end of the curve in Chart I (from 1902) to the point upon it corresponding with the year 1886, when the Returns are supposed to be fairly accurate, and if this line be then produced, it will be found to touch the highest portion of the mortality curve. The fall in the mortality from phthisis from the first year to the last is thus almost perfectly regular.

4. The male and female rates, when separated, also show a remarkable correspondence in their outlines, and testify to the general accuracy of the registration.

5. The simultaneous rise and fall of the rates in England, Scotland, and Ireland, presently to be noticed, point in the same direction.

It is mainly this singular regularity in the course of the disease which makes me venture to include the early as well as the later records in my survey. There may be, and probably are, inaccuracies in the Returns for individual years ; but, for the most part, these inaccuracies will be in defect, not in exaggeration of the phthisis-rate. It is more likely, for instance, that phthisis has been entered as bronchitis than that the converse has been the case. We may then, perhaps, accept the general outline of the curve as a fair representation of the truth. If this is so, and if the Charts are taken as delineating the actual course of the disease throughout the past 65 years, there are certain lessons which may be drawn from them.

A. *Periodic and Coincident Variations in the Phthisis-rate*

1. The first point to be noted is a tendency to periodicity in its prevalence. Phthisis is undoubtedly a communicable disease, but it is also endemic. It clings to certain localities, and, year by year, it persistently carries off large and similar percentages from the communities in which it prevails. Unlike the acute infectious complaints, such as scarlatina, measles, etc., it shows but little variation in its exactions from year to year, and pursues a comparatively steady course. As the several Charts show, it may, on the whole, as in Ireland, rise, or it may fall, as in England and Wales and Scotland ; but successive years display very little difference in the death-toll which it levies. There are, however, signs that even this chronic ailment is affected by widespread influences, such as meteorological conditions, and, possibly, that it may share with the more acute diseases the tendency to observe " periodic " times. From Chart I it appears that there were faint indications of a periodic rise in the disease in 1853, 1866, 1878, and 1890 ; and thus, if we begin to count from 1840, there are

five periods of from 12 to 13 years each. The indications are undoubtedly faint, but they may be sufficient to show that, as in the case of the acute exanthemata, there was, in the intervals of the periods, an accumulation of susceptible persons who had escaped the slighter infective influences, but who succumbed to the increased—almost epidemic—potency of the infection in these particular years : to the κατάστασις λοιμώδης as Hippocrates would have called it. This, however, is mere conjecture, and I do not lay any stress upon the occurrence.

2. It is evident, from the coincidences in the rise and fall of the disease in the three divisions of the kingdom, that there has been some widespread influence at work affecting the rate of mortality from phthisis.

(a) In the first place, there is a singular uniformity in the undulations of the male and female phthisis-rates in all three countries. In England and Wales (Chart II a), they rise and fall together in 89 per cent. of the years recorded, and only 11 are opposed in the directions of their course.

In Ireland (Chart IV), 73 per cent. are in the same direction, 24 per cent. in the opposite course, and 3 per cent. are neutral. In Scotland (Chart III), 83 per cent. are concurrent, and 17 are opposed.

In by far the majority of the years, therefore, there were conditions present which simultaneously raised or lowered the mortality from phthisis in the male and female populations respectively.

(b) Again, on comparing the English and Scotch curves, we find that, in 95 per cent. of the years in which there was any definite rise or fall, the two curves agreed. The English and Irish curves show about 80 per cent. of agreement ; the Scotch and Irish, 78 per cent. Obviously, the conditions influencing the mortality not only affected the two sexes, but they extended over the broad areas of Great Britain and Ireland.

(c) As might be almost assumed from the above-mentioned concurrences of the curves, the general contours of the lines are remarkably alike, especially in England and Scotland. In these countries they rise to their highest and sink to their lowest points, almost in the same years.

In Ireland the same tendency is to be observed, but owing to the general rise of the disease in that country, while it has been falling in England and Wales, it can only be noted in the lesser undulations of the curves[1]. We conclude, therefore, that there are widespread influences at work, extending over the whole of the British Isles, affecting both males and females, increasing or diminishing the death-rates from pulmonary tuberculosis.

It is natural, in the first instance, to turn to meteorological conditions for enlightenment as to the causes of the coincident variations in the death-rates, but the problem to be faced is an extremely difficult one.

In any attempt to compare our figures with the several elements of meteorology, we are met, firstly, by the extreme complexity of the conditions which make up what is called the "weather" of any given year; and secondly, by the impossibility of fixing the dates of origin of the mortal disease of which the termination only is recorded in the Tables.

The origin of acute diseases may often be brought into relation with certain of the meteorological elements, owing to their prevalence on certain dates; but in chronic ailments such as phthisis, the date on which the disease was contracted is always uncertain, and the fatal issue is usually separated by many months or years from the date of origin. The period of duration of the intervening illness is also so variable in different cases as to prevent any direct comparison between the heat or cold, the wetness or the dryness, of the year in which the complaint may have started.

It is highly probable, indeed, that certain states of the atmosphere may precipitate the fatal ending of even a chronic ailment, and that thus some slight perturbation in the course of the curve of disease might be produced which would point to its cause, if the weather returns and the death-rates were taken within sufficiently short periods of time. In this case, monthly, or even quarterly, returns would be likely to afford a basis for comparison better than annual returns.

Through the courtesy of the Mersey Docks and Harbour

[1] As I have already pointed out, these singular coincidences in the rise and fall of the disease in the three kingdoms are an additional proof of the general accuracy of the Returns.

Board, I have been supplied with interesting information respecting the weather in each year from 1867, and cordially thank them for the Tables now appended[1]. I have, however, been quite unable to trace any definite connection between the phthisis mortality and the weather, owing probably to the reasons which I have just given ; nothing in the temperature, in the wetness or dryness of the years, shows any distinct reason for the rise or fall of the disease curves. The solution of the problem must, therefore, be left to those who are better equipped for the research than I am.

B. *The Prospect of Abolishing Phthisis*

The next important lesson to be learnt from Chart I is a hopeful one. The total decline in the phthisis death-rate since the year 1838 is from over 3800 per million to 1100—a fall of over 70 per cent.—more than two-thirds reduction.

In a Paper read before the Epidemiological Society in 1896, entitled " Tuberculosis and Leprosy : A Parallel and a Prophecy " (see p. 190 of this volume), I ventured to call attention to this extraordinary decline in the death-rate from phthisis, and to compare it with that from leprosy. I then pointed out that, if phthisis diminished at about the same rate during another 30 years, it would have entirely disappeared by the end of that period.

Ten years have passed since then, and, although unfortunately the rate of diminution has somewhat slackened during this time, the phthisis-rate has fallen from 1400 to 1100 ; and we need only to amend our prophecy by extending the term of existence of the disease to the year 1930.

The last dregs of the poison will perhaps be difficult to cleanse away, but, unless sanitary progress is arrested, or some adverse circumstances arise in the interval, we may surely look for the almost total abolition of the disease in England by the middle of the present century.

C. *Causes of the Decline in the English Phthisis-rate*

When we study the course of phthisis mortality, as shown in Chart I, during the past 65 years, it becomes evident, from the

[1] Appendix I.

continuous steadiness of its decline, that it has not been due to any special measures of repression, but that there must have been some influences at work acting continuously throughout the whole period. Therefore, knowing what we do of the nature of tubercular infection, we must adopt one of the following conclusions : (1) that, during this period, the nation has gained increased power of resistance to infection ; (2) that there has been some impediment to the cultivation or growth of the specific germ ; or (3) that the microbe has been afforded fewer opportunities of attack. Probably all these several causes have been at work at the same time, and I think that we shall find that most of them may be grouped under the same head, as measures of sanitary reform.

When we look back, through the history of the last hundred years, for the first indication of a general sense of the value of sanitation, we find it most distinctly in the awakening of the nation after the terrible visitations of cholera and influenza in the years 1831, 1832 and 1833.

As Dr Chevers says, in his treatise *On Removable and Mitigable Causes of Death*, p. 40 : " The cholera of 1832 certainly had the effect of awakening the medical profession and conductors of the public press to the necessity of imitating our continental neighbours in their systems of public hygienic conservancy."

Truly, as he points out, " all that was proposed and achieved in England, expressly with a view to the preservation of the public health, antecedent to the present (nineteenth) century, might be comprised within a few sentences." It is true that he was able to point to a few legislative enactments on the subject in previous years, but nearly all the great sanitary reforms have taken place since the accession to the throne of our late good Queen Victoria.

Perhaps the most important of the earlier sanitary measures after 1832 was the institution of the Registrar-General's Returns of Births, Deaths, and Marriages in 1838. The revelations made by his earliest Reports, as to the enormous waste of life then proceeding in all our large towns, brought about the Health of Towns Commission, in 1842 ; and, shortly afterwards, steps were taken to mitigate their unhealthiness. Several towns appointed medical officers of health, notably Liverpool in 1847, and the City of London in 1848 ; and other towns soon followed their example.

In fact, the education of the public had begun, and a flood of literature from the pens of Dr W. Farr, Dr Southwood Smith, Mr Edwin Chadwick, and others, on sanitary reform, soon took effect on the minds of the more thoughtful of the people, and the country began to attempt to cleanse its Augean stable.

In 1845, laws were passed containing regulations respecting buildings, their drainage and ventilation, and this was soon followed by others in the same direction. In 1848, the first Public Health Act was passed ; also the laws against the sale of diseased meat, and other beneficent measures followed, such as the abolition of the Window Tax, in 1851.

All this activity in the cause of the public health must have had an effect, not only on the general death-rate, but also on the phthisis-rate, though no idea was entertained at the time that this disease was at least as preventable as many others. We are now better able to understand the results of this unconscious campaign against phthisis ; and it may be worth while to indicate the modes in which the several sanitary measures acted in reducing the hitherto heavy mortality from tubercular diseases.

1. *Ventilation.* At the present day, no one can doubt the close relation that exists between " re-breathed air " and phthisis. It has been established by a thousand proofs, and need not here be elaborated. It may be explained, however, in several ways : (1) by the greater frequency in such air of the specific germ of the disease ; (2) by the long life of the bacillus of tubercle in the presence of the aqueous vapour of the breath[1] ; (3) by the co-existence of other pathogenic organisms, which prepare the way for, or hasten the action of, the specific disease ; (4) by the pre-disposition to the disease which such air produces, either by lowering the natural resistance of the body, or by inducing diseases which open the way for the bacillus of tubercle ; (5) lastly, to the fact that such air is most found where other sanitary defects, such as bad drainage and little sunlight are present ; where the most delicate and otherwise diseased populations are to be found, and where intemperance and other evils are likely to assist the attack of the micro-organism.

---

[1] See p. 23 of *Researches on Tuberculosis*, Weber-Parkes Prize Essay, 1897, by the writer (Smith, Elder and Co.), and Paper 6, Sect. III. in this volume.

Whatever the explanation, the Registrar-General's Reports, and the other annals of public health, teem with instances of the evil effects of respiratory impurity, especially in engendering tubercular disease, and of the immediate amelioration produced by free ventilation.

It has already been pointed out that, even anterior to the year 1832, some attempts at sanitation had been made; and among these measures must be classed the efforts, in the middle of the eighteenth century, to obtain better ventilation of ships and of public buildings.

Early in the eighteenth century, Pringle pointed out that the air of the military hospitals killed more than the sword. " Plus occidit aer quam gladius "; and he called in the assistance of skilled mechanicians to improve their ventilation. It was at his request that, in 1726, trial was made in the House of Commons of a centrifugal fan; and, a few years afterwards, we are told that as many as 20 Reports on the subject had been laid before the House. Before this, the better ventilation of the ships of the British Navy had been carried out; and about the same time the heavy infantile death-rate at the Rotunda Hospital, Dublin, had been greatly diminished by the introduction of improved methods of ventilation. Other hospitals and public buildings soon followed these examples; and we cannot doubt that the public mind was turned in this direction, and that people were becoming alive to the danger of breathing air fouled with respiratory impurity Probably these facts will account for at least a part of the diminished rates of mortality from consumption before the year 1836[1].

2. *Land Drainage.* Another important sanitary measure was also partially set to work in Great Britain before the great period of sanitary reform—I mean, land-drainage on a large scale. This was no doubt done with a view to the interests of agriculture; but, incidentally, it put a stop to malarial disease in the Fen country, and we may be sure that it also affected the phthisis mortality.

---

[1] It is interesting to observe that, about this time, Dr Franklin, the famous American, was accustomed to take what were then called " air baths," and it was proposed to use them medicinally (*Dict. des Sciences Medicales*, Paris, 1820, Art. " Ventilation," p. 167).

Extensive systems of sewerage were also established in many large towns early in the century, and sewage commissioners were appointed ; and the drying of the soil which resulted, not only lowered the general death-rates of the places concerned, but, to the astonishment of many sanitarians, diminished greatly the phthisis-rates of most of the towns thus improved.

Commenting upon Dr Buchanan's account of the results of " improved drainage and water-supply " (in 1866), Sir John Simon remarks[1] that " the novel and most important conclusion suggests itself, that *the drying of soil, which has in most cases accompanied the laying of main sewers in the improved towns, has led to the diminution, more or less considerable, of phthisis.*"

As we know, Dr Buchanan continued his researches ; and, in an inquiry into the distribution of phthisis on impervious and porous soils, he confirmed his observations and, without knowing it, those also of Dr Bowditch, of Massachusetts, that phthisis is most rife on impervious, undrained soils. A few years later, the Registrar-General for Scotland also corroborated the facts as stated.

After giving a list of 15 towns in which phthisis had thus been diminished, Sir John Simon observes : " the fact that, in some of these cases, the diminished fatality of phthisis is by far the largest amendment, if not the only one which has taken place in the local health, becomes extremely interesting and significant, when the circumstance is remembered that works of sewerage, by which the drying of soil is effected, must always of necessity precede the accomplishment of other objects (house-drainage, abolition of cesspools, and so forth) on which the cessation of various other diseases is dependent."

I do not think that this singular influence of dry subsoils in preventing phthisis has ever been fully explained ; but, accepting the fact as we must, I am now inclined to trace a considerable part of the decline in the earlier portions of the phthisis-curve in England to the general and special drainage works which were actively carried out about this time.

3. *The Sanitary Improvement of Dwellings.* The most potent of all the means which have hitherto been unconsciously employed

---

[1] *Ninth Report to the Privy Council.*

for the suppression of phthisis is the improvement of dwellings, and especially of artizans' and labourers' dwellings.

In a Paper read before the Epidemiological Society on May 11, 1887, on "Tubercular Infective Areas," I pointed out the fact that tubercular infection clings to certain houses, and even to certain unhealthy areas ; and this observation has also been made by Dr Flick, of Philadelphia, Dr Niven, of Manchester, and others.

Moreover, researches, pursued by myself, in conjunction with Professors Dreschfeld and Delépine, of Manchester, proved that tubercular sputum would live for months in a small, badly-drained, ill-ventilated cottage in Ancoats : whilst it was speedily deprived of all virulence in a healthy dwelling on a dry, sandy soil.

The observations of Dr Russell, of Glasgow, and others, on the prevalence of phthisis in one-roomed tenements, as compared with the better classes of dwellings, show strongly the influence of the home upon the disease.

It would not be surprising, therefore, to find that the many Acts which have been passed since 1848 had resulted in a great diminution of the mortality from phthisis. Most large towns have also secured private Acts, by means of which " rookeries " have been abolished, unhealthy areas have been cleared, and healthy dwellings erected in their stead. Beyond all this, the Building Byelaws of some enlightened communities, such as London and Liverpool, have secured the adequate entrance of light, as well as air, into streets. Wherever all this has been done, we find a great improvement in the health of the inhabitants, and especially a smaller proportion of deaths from tubercular disease. We cannot doubt that much of the obvious decline and fall of this mortality, in the middle and end of the last century, has been due to these improvements in the sanitary conditions of the dwellings of the poor.

4. *The Amelioration of Social Conditions.* We cannot, however, claim all this diminution of mortality as due to purely sanitary reforms. It seems certain that the resistance of the population to infection must have been increased by means of the better food, and better clothing, and more healthy environment, that became possible after the Repeal of the Corn Laws in 1847, and by the subsequent adoption of the principle of free imports into the country.

We might perhaps expect, therefore, to find some evidence of this fact in a further and more rapid decline of the curves of mortality from phthisis. There is, however, nothing very decisive to note on this point. It is true that there is a somewhat rapid decline of the curve after 1847 ; but we must remember that food did not at once become cheaper until some little time after the cessation of the duties ; and again, that most of the cases of the disease which ended fatally in 1847 must have commenced many months before that date. Moreover, there is again a rapid rise in the mortality four years later, in 1851, so that we can hardly claim the preceding descent as evidence of greater resisting power.

During the Cotton Famine, from 1863 to 1866, there is a decided rise in the curve, as if the privations of that time had been able to destroy a certain number of the more weakly individuals ; but the curve again descends rapidly after 1866, thus showing that no permanent injury had been done to the workpeople.

Again, after 1870, when the prosperity of the country was said to be " advancing by leaps and bounds," there is a great drop in the mortality, but it is not possible to differentiate it from the improvement that was evidently going on owing to other sanitary reforms which have already been noticed. We must be satisfied to group all these beneficent influences together, and note their combined effect.

This is one view of the progress of social reforms which' have been favourable to the public health and hostile to the bacillus of tubercle. On the other hand, it is certain that some social conditions which are likely to add to the danger of infection by the organism have become greatly aggravated during the period in question. Thus, a much larger proportion of the population have come from country districts into towns. Most of these people, also, both males and females, have gradually drifted into the most crowded and least healthy parts of these towns ; and, in place of wholesome outdoor work, they have taken to indoor occupations in, for the most part, badly-ventilated workplaces, and their leisure time is usually spent in unhealthy surroundings.

Consider, for instance, the sort of life which a healthy country lad is likely to lead when he migrates into a town. He probably takes up his abode in a " common lodging-house," where his next bedfellow may be consumptive, and where the spitting habits of the whole community scatter filth and infection broadcast. He obtains work in some place where the atmosphere is polluted with similar material, and where dusts of all kinds are ready to prepare the way for the specific organism to enter his lungs and dwell there. In the evening, he perhaps goes to some dirty, badly-ventilated music-hall, or to the pit of a theatre, where again the air he breathes is contaminated with much tubercular matter; or he may go with his mates to a public-house, and sit there for hours in at least equally unhealthy surroundings. It is, surely, not surprising that many of these young males should contract, and die of, phthisis.

The influence of the common lodging-house in spreading phthisis is very grievous. Thus Dr Niven, in his admirable Report upon these places, presented to the Manchester Corporation in 1899, says (at p. 5): " There is one disease—viz. consumption—which does not need to be introduced, being already in possession, which plays great havoc amongst the inhabitants of common lodging-houses." From 77 such houses in the Angel Meadow district, containing an average population of 1825 persons, the death-registers furnished, in the years 1893–95, 110 deaths from phthisis, giving an annual death-rate from the disease of over 20 per thousand during that period.

" Nor is the mischief confined to the inhabitants of these houses. The consumptive labourers, hawkers, joiners, bakers, butchers, tailors, mechanics, clerks, washerwomen, will not only give the disease to their workmates who do not live in common lodging-houses, but may in some employments convey it to those who purchase the goods they are engaged in making or vending. Moreover, they will certainly disseminate it in the district in which they live."

Take the case, again, of a female immigrant into a large town. She is pretty sure to drift into some unsanitary " slum," or into a dirty, overcrowded lodging. She takes work in a dusty, ill-ventilated factory, or she marries early and lives in a tenement-house, or in a dwelling all of whose windows are shut in order to keep out the outer air, polluted as it is with " smuts " and other impurities. Her chief amusements are gossiping in similar houses to her own, and an occasional visit to dusty, hot, and close music-halls. On the other hand, she may be devout, and may spend some time in dark and badly-ventilated chapels or churches; but in all these places she constantly runs the risk of tubercular infection. These are all reasons for an increase, instead of a diminution, in phthisis mortality; and if it were not for the enormous improvements which we have seen to have taken place of late in the sanitary condition of our large towns, the great immigration into them of young males and females must have led to this result.

As matters are now, however, the conditions of life in our country villages are often worse than those in towns, and they only escape a larger phthisis-rate owing to the smaller volume of infective material and to the sparseness of their populations.

5. *Temperance.* The question of the relative sobriety of the populations at different epochs has from two points of view an important bearing upon our subject : (1) because of the predisposition to the disease produced by intemperate habits; and (2) because of the facilities for infection met with in the places frequented by drunkards.

It is somewhat difficult to estimate the exact amount of growth of temperance throughout the nation. On the one hand, from ordinary observation, it would appear that there really is less drunkenness now, in most classes of society, than there was 50 or 60 years ago. It is certainly so in the upper classes; and the movement in favour of temperance has spread widely in the Navy and Army, and, to some extent, among the working classes.

On the other hand, from Mulhall's statistics, quoted by Dr Niven, in his paper " On the Economics of Health," it may be shown that very little change has taken place since 1853 in the consumption of beer and spirits per head of the population; so that, if there is less drunkenness, the use of alcohol must be more widely spread among the people, and the public-house continues to be, perhaps, more than ever the " Club of the Working Man."

Of the two factors, then, one, inebriety, may have diminished; and, if so, this diminution can hardly fail to have had an influence upon the phthisis-mortality. There will now be fewer drunkards, predisposed to consumption by their habits of life; fewer drunkards' homes, in which the seeds of the disease might have been sown in the rising generation; fewer neglected children to carry on the infection.

But if, on the other hand, the public-house has not lost its hold on both the idlers and the workers of the population, then, even though there be less drunkenness, a most potent breeding-ground of the disease is left, and its influence is shown in the excess of male phthisis-mortality.

There is, however, a possible source of fallacy which should be taken into account in our reasoning on this and other statistical points in relation to this subject.

Dr Niven has pointed out to me the fact that, of late years, there has been a distinct alteration in the numbers of the population in the different " age groups "; that the number of young persons at ages little affected by phthisis, *e.g.* between 0 and 15, has diminished proportionately to the number of those at ages more prone to the disease : *i.e.* from 15 to 45. This change in the constitution of the population would naturally tend to increase the phthisis-rate per million. This simple cause will, therefore, to some extent explain the slackening of the downward tendency of the curve, but it will not cover the whole ground. If it were the sole influence at work, it would certainly affect both the male and the female rates. But, as we can see in Chart II, the female rate shows very little alteration in its rate of descent. It is the mortality among males that chiefly raises the curve of mortality of persons of both sexes in Chart I.

On the whole, I am inclined to think that, in the last 30 years, habits of temperance have not availed to stem the stream of infection flowing from the other social habits of the working classes; and that, so far, they have done but little to diminish the mortality from phthisis.

6. *Notification, Disinfection, and Isolation.* Hitherto we have not had to record any special methods for the repression of the disease. Phthisis was indeed recognised as to some extent a " preventable disease, " by such masters of sanitary science as Dr W. Farr and Sir John Simon ; but, beyond recommendations of better ventilation of barracks, workplaces, etc., and of the provision of lung-spaces in towns, and of better drainage of districts, no direct effort was made to prevent the communication of the disease.

No such means of disinfection as was practised in Italy and the south of France, for instance, was ever used.

Consumption was indeed regarded as an infectious disease by many physicians long before the discovery of the bacillus of tubercle. It was impossible that it should have been otherwise, after the researches of Villemin, in 1865, and of other pathologists shortly afterwards. It may be safely said, however, that no practical attempts were made to prevent infection, until Koch pointed out the danger arising from tuberculous dust, and Cornet found the specific organism on the walls of rooms that had been occupied by phthisical patients.

I believe that one of the first attempts at organised voluntary notification of phthisis and disinfection of houses in England was made at my suggestion by the medical staffs of the Consumption Hospital and of the Royal Infirmary in Manchester, in the year 1892. At a meeting of these gentlemen, which was also attended by Dr Tatham, then Medical Officer of Health for Manchester, a scheme was drawn up, and, thanks to the public spirit and energy of Dr Tatham, it was at once put into practice, and was continued for several months. It was then abandoned for a time, in order that Prof. Delépine might make experiments upon the efficiency of the methods of disinfection employed. The work in Manchester was afterwards independently and thoroughly carried out by Dr Niven, upon a system of his own, originally formulated in Oldham, but extended and revised to meet the requirements of the Manchester City Council. About the same time (in 1893–4) an admirable system of dealing with infected persons and infected houses was carried out in New York, and various towns in England and Scotland followed these examples.

In 1895, the National Association for the Prevention of Tuberculosis was established under the Presidency of the Prince of Wales ; and it has done much to call public attention to the danger of infection, and to the means of warding off the disease.

During the last few years, also, numerous sanatoria for the reception of consumptive patients have been established, and their reports claim a large measure of success in combating the complaint. Altogether it may be said that, within the last decade, a fairly strong direct effort has been made to abolish consumption.

It might have been anticipated that such an active campaign against the disease would result in some noteworthy reduction in the phthisis mortality. It is disconcerting, therefore, to find that although the curve of the disease still declines on the whole, yet it falls at a diminished rate. There is even a slight rise from 1896 to 1900, and in the latter year its rate is nearly as high as it was in 1895. It falls again in the three following years, but no faster than it did from 1890 to 1895. As I have already pointed out, also, this slackening in the rate of descent cannot be due to the alteration in the grouping of the population, as it is confined to the curve of the male mortality. On the whole, I think that it must be admitted that there is something to be explained in regard to this apparent arrest in the fall of the phthisis-rate.

It cannot be supposed that the direct measures of repression which we have just passed under review have had no effect; nor can we admit that there has been any slackening in the energy with which general sanitary reforms have been carried out. I have made careful inquiries on this point in London, Liverpool, and Manchester, and in all these places the female rates have been steadily diminishing, especially in Liverpool (Chart V), where most active work of reconstruction of unhealthy areas has been going on for many years. The male rate always lags behind that of the females, and is throughout the greater.

From returns kindly furnished to me by Professor Hope, of Liverpool, and by Dr Niven, of Manchester, I have drawn the Charts (Nos. V and VI)—which show the variations in the male and female phthisis-mortality for a number of years. In each of these cities I am informed that from 6000 to 7000 unsanitary dwellings have been dealt with[1]. The power of sanitary reform,

---

[1] Since the reading of this Paper, Sir Shirley F. Murphy has kindly furnished me with the male and female phthisis-rates for London, from 1851 to 1903. These figures are uncorrected for institutions, but are sufficiently correct for our purpose, as will be seen by comparing the uncorrected with the corrected rates for the years 1895 to 1903. Time does not permit charts to be made from these figures, but they are given *in extenso* in an Appendix. They will clearly show that similar conditions to those in Liverpool and Manchester are found in London. There is the same preponderance of male over female deaths. The descent of the female rate is also more decided and more rapid than that of the males.

then, in mitigating the disease among females is therein made clearly evident, but among males it is obvious that it has had less effect.

From the consideration of these facts we are almost driven to conclude that some malign influence has intervened to prevent both the sets of agencies mentioned from having their full effect upon the males of the population. In other words, that there must be some permanent sources of infection which, at the present time, are out of reach of these beneficent agencies. Now, when we look around for sources of infection mainly affecting males, there are three which stand prominently forward :

1. The imperfect ventilation of many of the workplaces in which both sexes are employed, but in which the spitting habits of the males expose them to greater danger than the females.

2. The habitual use of common lodging-houses, which is more prevalent among men than women. This source of danger has already been alluded to.

3. The constant resort of the working-man to the public-house, and his long-continued sitting and inhaling of the sputum-laden air.

I have already mentioned this last source of infection as a cause of the still untouched residuum of tubercular disease. We shall find further grounds for this opinion in the next section.

D. *Causes of the Differences between the Phthisis-rates of England Scotland, and Ireland*

Hitherto, in our contemplation of Charts II (*a*), III, and IV, we have dwelt mainly upon the singular coincidences to be found between the minor undulations of the curves. We have now to consider their equally remarkable differences and their significance.

These differences are chiefly three :

1. The deplorable fact that, whilst in England and Scotland the phthisis-mortality has greatly diminished, in Ireland it has increased by about one-fourth, in the course of the 37 years recorded by the Registrar-General.

2. We have the strange circumstance that, whilst in Scotland and Ireland the female rate exceeds the male, in England the reverse is the case.

3. In both England and Scotland, the female rate descends more rapidly than the male.

These facts need explanation ; and in attempting to account for them, I think that we shall find some corroboration of the conclusions at which we have arrived as to the variations in the English phthisis-rate.

With regard to the increased phthisis mortality in Ireland, it is most probable that it is due mainly to the absence—in the greater portion of the country—of those beneficial sanitary reforms which we have found to be such potent weapons against tubercular disease.

Although in one or two towns a certain degree of sanitary effort has been made, it is incontestable that all over the country sanitation, such as we have been accustomed to in England and Scotland, has not been carried out. The greater part of the country is still undrained ; the hovels in which the peasantry used to live and die are hovels still ; cleanliness is rare, and nuisances of all kinds abound to almost as great an extent as they did formerly. In Dublin and many other towns, there are an abundance of breeding-places for the tubercle bacillus.

The Report of the Royal Commission on Towns in Ireland, in 1877, says that : " revelations of a very startling and shocking nature were brought before us, indicating an almost culpable degree of apathy on the part alike of the sanitary authorities and the inhabitants[1]."

Sir J. W. Moore also tells us that " the Sanitary Act of 1877 was so faulty and so stingy in its provisions for the payment of the Medical Officers of Health, that sanitation in Ireland has received a check, which, even if public opinion is gradually brought to bear upon the subject, 20 years will scarcely remedy[2]."

We can hardly doubt that this neglect of sanitary reform has withheld from Ireland many of the beneficent measures which in England have proved so powerful in restraining tubercular disease.

We must add to these adverse influences the fact that owing to the excessive emigration from Ireland of many of the most able-bodied and healthy persons of both sexes, a large proportionate

---

[1] Quoted by Sir J. W. Moore, in an Address on State Medicine in 1885.
[2] *Dublin Journal of Medical Science*, vol. LXXIX. p. 212.

residuum of weakly and tubercularly-susceptible individuals have been left behind, to run the gauntlet of infective agencies, fostered by the neglect of sanitary measures.

Here again, however, we must point out that this influence would affect both males and females.

It would also surely have had most effect in the early years of the period, when the exodus of the population was most manifest.

It has further been suggested to me by Mr W. J. Crossley, that some part of the increased mortality from phthisis in Ireland may be due to the fact that now buttermilk is much less used in the ordinary diet of the peasant than it was formerly.

The " Creameries " that have been established throughout the country take most of the milk, and export it in various forms, so that this source of nourishment has been greatly diminished.

On the whole, then, we must conclude that the main causes of the rise in the Irish phthisis-rates of both males and females are to be found in the want of proper ventilation of dwellings, in the lack of land drainage, in the want of healthy environment, and especially the dampness of the surroundings ; in the lack of proper nourishment, in habits of intemperance, and, lastly, in the imperfect manner in which the direct means of combating the infection have been carried out. Many of the above-mentioned causes of the disease would fall most heavily upon the female population, and hence probably arises the predominance of the female over the male rates of mortality.

The adverse influences mainly affecting males in England have already been indicated, namely, the practice of spitting in ill-ventilated workplaces, common lodging-houses, and the public-house. Owing to these causes, while the female rate has been lowered more than one-half in 28 years (from 2113 to 993), the male rate has gone down less than one-third (from 2296 to 1427). But another point has also to be noted, namely, that throughout the whole period for which the figures are available in England, whilst the above-mentioned adverse circumstances have been able to keep the male rate above the female rate, a complete contrast to this state of affairs is to be found in Ireland and Scotland ; in these countries—except at the very end of the period—the female rate is the higher of the two. It would be interesting if some explanation could be given of this difference. Probably some part of it is due to the different degrees to which the several populations are attracted to indoor employments.

Dr Greenhow was the first to point out (in 1868) that, in proportion as workpeople were occupied in indoor employments, so did the mortality from lung disease increase ; if more males than females were so employed their rate was higher and *vice versa*. His observations on this point have been amply confirmed by others.

According to this rule we should expect the female rate to be usually the higher, as women more commonly work indoors, often at home, in household occupations. This is so, even in England, in the agricultural counties, where the female rate of mortality from phthisis exceeds the male rate. But in this country, so great is the power of the adverse circumstances which have been mentioned, that, as we have seen, the total phthisis-rates of the males constantly exceed those of the females, and their grade of decent is less abrupt. In Ireland and Scotland, however, where the men mostly work out of doors, it is the women who suffer most from the disease. Are, then, the malign influences less potent in these countries than in England ? An inquiry into the differences in the habits of the several populations might throw some light upon this question.

Looking broadly at the matter, it seems clear that there are certain differences in some of their habits. Thus, in Ireland and Scotland, although the peoples are for the most part of different religions, yet they are, especially the females, more inclined to attend divine service in church or chapel than are the bulk of English people ; and these places of worship are notoriously badly ventilated. On the other hand, the English, especially the males, are more inclined to all kinds of social gatherings in equally badly-ventilated rooms. Again, although the spitting habit may be equally common among the males of all three countries, this source of infection is more likely to affect the Englishman than either the Scotchman or the Irishman. There is but little desecration of church or chapel by spitting on the floors, the women using their handkerchiefs for this purpose ; but it is notorious how

general is this disgusting habit in most of the places frequented
by the English working-man.

In each of the three sources of infection which we have mentioned as the cause of the excessive mortality of the English
workman, it is the tuberculous dust spread by this habit which is
the main agent at work : in the workplace, in the common
lodging-house, and in the public-house.

Although I am not well acquainted with the habits of the
Scotch or Irish in this respect, yet I should suppose that it would
at least be less hurtful to them than it is to the Englishman.

Owing to his prevailing occupations, the Irishman and the
Scotchman would mostly spit out of doors ; the Englishman
indoors on the floor of any place where he might be. The drinking
habits of the three nations may also tend towards this result.
Although they may, on the average, take about the same amount
of alcohol per person, they take it, for the most part, in different
fashions. The Scotchman goes into his " dram-shop," quickly
drinks down his dram, and goes out again immediately. The
Irishman often does the same, though he may perhaps linger for a
longer time, taking his porter or his " toddy " in sips ; but we
know how long an English labourer sits in the bar or tap-room,
drinking successive glasses of beer, treating his friends, and discussing the affairs of his parish or of the nation. A tuberculous
person spits as freely upon the floor as his healthy neighbour, and
the tuberculous matter dries up amongst the sand or sawdust,
gets ground into a fine powder, and when swept up flies into the
air on wings of epithelium, and so is ready to lodge in any susceptible person's lungs. I believe that these differing circumstances
will account for most of the differences in the phthisis-rates of the
three kingdoms.

E. *The further Campaign against Phthisis*

There are several lessons to be learnt from this review of phthisis-
mortality, especially in regard to the future campaign against this
disease.

Thus (1), although so far the direct measures of repression,
such as notification and disinfection, have been overweighted by

adverse circumstances, and have made no apparent impression upon the rates of mortality, yet we cannot doubt that ultimately they must have an effect, and must be energetically persevered with, especially the disinfection of houses in which phthisical patients have lived or died.

But (2) we cannot forget that, however closely the net of notification may be drawn around the known consumptives, a large number will nevertheless escape through its meshes, and will spread the specific infection broadcast. Accordingly, it will always be necessary to use the other means of quelling the disease which have proved so efficacious in the past. We must, therefore, persevere with all the measures of sanitary reform, which act by removing the chief conditions under which alone infection becomes possible. We have seen that even when the seeds of this infection were present in large quantities, yet free ventilation, good drainage, sunshine, and abundance of good food and clothing, have reduced the phthisis mortality of males in England by nearly two-thirds, and of females by nearly three-quarters. It would, therefore, be folly to give up the weapons which have already produced so magnificent a result, and trust only to the continental methods of isolation and disinfection.

Much as has been done, much more yet remains to be done, in the way of opening up the blind streets and alleys in our large towns, the destruction of insanitary property, the building and proper management of healthy dwellings of the poor, and the preservation of as pure an atmosphere as possible in all communities of human beings. More persistent efforts will also have to be made to obtain herds of tubercle-free cattle throughout the country. When all this is accomplished, however, I fear that there will still remain the adverse influences which we have seen to weigh so heavily, especially upon the male phthisis-rates.

If we are to clear away the last dregs of the disease from the population of these islands, it will be necessary to adopt stringent measures against the spitting habit in all public places, and also in workplaces, common lodging-houses, and public bars and tap-rooms. Moreover, efficient ventilation must be established by law in all these places, and also in all places of public assembly : in theatres, concert-rooms, churches and chapels ; and, not only

air, but adequate light, must also be admitted. The education of
the public, and especially of the children, in general hygiene and
in the best methods of avoiding tuberculosis infection, must be
more adequately carried out. When all this has been accomplished
we might then hope to see a steady and more rapid descent of the
phthisis-mortality curve, and might expect that, after not many
decades of years, this opprobrium of our race will cease to exist.

The Appendices to this Paper will be found on pages 256–59.

APPENDIX I. MERSEY DOCKS AND HARBOUR BOARD

LIVERPOOL OBSERVATORY, BIDSTON, BIRKENHEAD

General Character of the Weather for the Years 1867 to 1903 inclusive

Year	Rain	Cloudiness	Temperature	Wind	
				Velocity	Direction
1867	Below average	Cloudy	Average	Below average	S.E. and W.
1868	Below average	Very bright	Above average	Above average	S.W. and N.W.
1869	Above average	Bright	Average	Average	S.W. and N.W.
1870	Much below average	Very bright	Below average	Below average	S.W. and S.E
1871	Below average	Average	Above average	Average	S.E. and S.W.
1872	Abnormal, 45·664 ins.	Cloudy	Above average	Average	S.E. and S.W.
1873	Much below average	Cloudy	Average	Above average	S. and S.W.
1874	Below average	Cloudy	Average	Above average	S.W. and N.W.
1875	Average	Cloudy	Average	Much below average	S.E and S.W.
1876	Slightly above average	Bright	Average	Above average	S.E. and S.W.
1877	Much above average	Very cloudy	Average	Average	S.E. and S.W.
1878	Little below average	Cloudy	Average	Below average	S. and N.W.
1879	Average	Very cloudy	Much below average	Above average	S.E. and S.W.
1880	Above average	Cloudy	Average	Much below average	S.E. and S.W.
1881	Above average	Cloudy	Below average	Above average	S.E. and S.W.
1882	Above average	Fairly bright	Average	Above average	S.E. and S.W.
1883	Below average	Cloudy	Below average	Average	S.W. and N.W.
1884	Below average	Very bright	Above average	Much below average	S.E. and S.W.

Year					
1885	Average	Bright	Below average	Slightly below average	S.E. and S.W.
1886	Above average	Fairly bright	Below average	Much below average	S.E. and S.W.
1887	Much below average	Very bright	Below average	Slightly below average	S.W. and N.W.
1888	Much below average	Very cloudy	Below average	Above average	S.E. and W.
1889	Little below average	Very cloudy	Below average	Average	S.E. and W.
1890	Little below average	Very cloudy	Below average	Above average	S.E. and S.W.
1891	Above average	Very cloudy	Below average	Average	E. and S.W.
1892	Above average	Very cloudy	Above average	Above average	S.E. and W
1893	Above average	Very bright	Above average	Above average	S.E. and W.
1894	Little below average	Fairly bright	Above average	Average	S. and W.
1895	Little below average	Fairly bright	Below average	Above average	S.E. and W.
1896	Little below average	Cloudy	Slightly above average	Average	S.E. and W.
1897	Average	Cloudy	Average	Above average	S.E. and N.W.
1898	Below average	Cloudy	Above average	Average	S.S.E. and S.W.
1899	Below average	Fairly bright	Slightly above average	Below average	S.E. and W.
1900	Above average	Very cloudy	Slightly above average	Above average	S.E. and S.W.
1901	Above average	Fairly bright	Average	Average	S.E. and W.
1902	Below average	Cloudy	Below average	Above average	E. and N.W.
1903	Above average	Cloudy	Average	Above average	S.E. and N.W

APPENDIX I. *Continued*

*Statement of Mean Maximum and Mean Minimum Air Temperatures
taken at* 9 A.M. *daily from* 1867 *to* 1903, *inclusive*

	Air Temperature			Air Temperature	
Year	Mean Maximum	Mean Minimum	Year	Mean Maximum	Mean Minimum
	Deg.	Deg.		Deg.	Deg.
1867	54·7	43·2	1886	53·1	43·3
1868	57·4	44·9	1887	53·4	42·6
1869	55·5	44·1	1888	52·8	42·7
1870	54·9	43·1	1889	50·4	43·8
1871	54·9	43·2	1890	53·9	43·7
1872	56·0	44·4	1891	53·6	42·9
1873	54·0	43·5	1892	52·6	42·4
1874	54·9	44·0	1893	56·7	45·0
1875	54·2	44·3	1894	55·1	44·4
1876	54·5	43·9	1895	53·4	42·6
1877	54·2	44·2	1896	54·6	44·1
1878	54·4	44·6	1897	54·6	44·1
1879	50·9	41·7	1898	55·5	45·1
1880	54·2	44·1	1899	55·2	44·2
1881	52·8	42·5	1900	54·3	44·4
1882	54·4	44·4	1901	54·3	43·7
1883	53·9	44·0	1902	53·1	43·3
1884	56·4	44·9	1903	53·9	44·1
1885	52·8	42·9			

APPENDIX II.   ADMINISTRATIVE COUNTY OF LONDON
                (SIR SHIRLEY F. MURPHY)

PHTHISIS.   *Death-rates per* 1000 *living,* 1851 *to* 1903

Year	Males	Females	Year	Males	Females
1851	3·459	2·538	1878	3·054	2·156
1852	3·330	2·566	1879	3·001	1·995
1853	3·462	2·603	1880	2·705	1·839
1854	3·337	2·510	1881	2·687	1·846
1855	3·410	2·648	1882	2·714	1·801
1856	3·152	2·519	1883	2·749	1·857
1857	3·229	2·416	1884	2·701	1·798
1858	3·162	2·420	1885	2·536	1·712
1859	3·329	2·436	1886	2·571	1·663
1860	3·224	2·417	1887	2·363	1·541
1861	3·224	2·359	1888	2·275	1·438
1862	3·177	2·380	1889	2·371	1·436
1863	3·110	2·376	1890	2·622	1·591
1864	3·474	2·482	1891	2·480	1·512
1865	3·419	2·476	1892	2·320	1·415
1866	3·705	2·589	1893	2·340	1·439
1867	3·446	2·407	1894	2·179	1·283
1868	3·411	2·386	1895	2·219	1·374
1869	3·284	2·331	1896	2·159	1·296
1870	3·349	2·275	1897	2·242	1·281
1871	3·116	2·256	1898	2·274	1·275
1872	3·118	2·121	1899	2·378	1·370
1873	3·042	2·163	1900	2·270	1·224
1874	3·000	2·034	1901	2·145	1·186
1875	3·152	2·174	1902	2·089	1·107
1876	3·112	2·139	1903	2·011	1·089
1877	2·944	2·041			

PHTHISIS.   *Death-rates per* 1000 *living*

Year	Death-rate[1] not fully corrected for Institutions	Death-rate[2] fully corrected for Institutions
1895	1·83	1·77
1896	1·73	1·68
1897	1·78	1·71
1898	1·79	1·72
1899	1·90	1·82
1900	1·79	1·73
1901	1·71	1.66
1902	1·64	1·60
1903	1·60	1·55

[1] Including deaths of Londoners in the Metropolitan workhouses, hospitals and lunatic asylums outside the County of London, but excluding deaths of non-Londoners in the Willesden Workhouse, the London Fever Hospital, the Metropolitan Asylums Board's Hospitals, and the Middlesex County Lunatic Asylum, within the County of London.

[2] These death-rates are fully corrected for institutions, *i.e.* by the exclusion of deaths of persons not belonging to but occurring in institutions situated within London, and by the inclusion of deaths of persons belonging to London, but occurring in London institutions situate outside the Administrative County.

INDEX